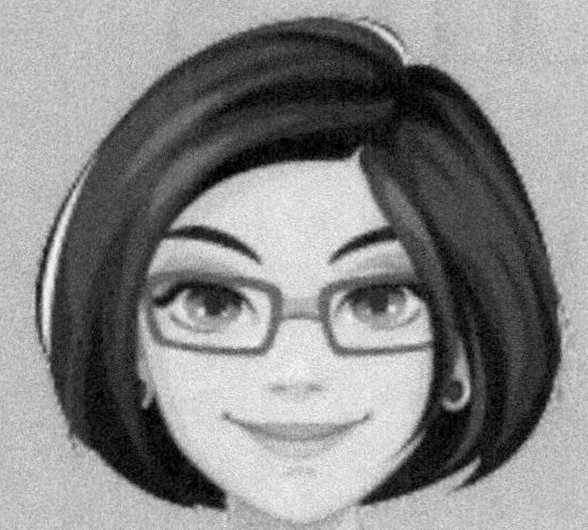

NURSING MNEMONICS

Memory Tricks to Crush the Nursing School and Trigger Your Nursing Memory

163 Mnemonics	Flashcards	Quiz
Test	Word Search	Crosswords
Matching	Table Review	

Mnemonics
Table Review

nursing, mnemonics,acronym,

Question	Answer
Steps in the Nursing Process ADPIE (A Delicious PIE)	A-ssessment D- iagnosis P-lanning I-mplementation E-valuaton
Steps in the Nursing Process AAPIE (An Apple Pie)	A-ssessment A-nanlysis P-lanning I-mplementation E-valuation
Inflammation (HIPER)	H-eat I-nduration P-ain E-dema R-edness
Acid-Base (ROME)	R-espiratory O-pposite M-etabolic E-qual
CANCER'S Early Warning Signs CAUTION UP	Change in bowel/bladder A lesion doesn't heal Unusual bleeding/discharge Thickening lump in breast/elsewhere Indigestion/difficulty swallowing Obvious changes wart/mole Nagging cough/persistent hoarseness Unexplained weight loss Pernicious Anemia
CANCER Interventions	C-omfort A-ltered Body Image N-utrition C-hemotherapy E-valuate response to meds R-espite for caretakers
Hypoglycemia (TIRED) - an abnormal decrease of blood in the sugar	T-achycardia I-rritability R-estless E-xcessive Hunger D-iaphoresis/ Depression
Adrenal Gland Hormones (SSS)	S-ugar (Glucocorticoids) S-alt (Mineralcorticoids) S-ex (Androgens)
Pulmonary Edema (MAD DOG)	M-Morphine A-Aminophylline D- Digitalis D-Diuretics (Lasix) O- Oxygen G-ases (Blood Gases ABG's)
5 P's of Circulatory Checks	P-Pain P-Paresthesia P-Paralysis P-Pulse P-Pallor (Paleness)
Hypertension Nursing Care (DIURETIC)	D-aily Weight I- ntake and Output (I & O) U- rine Output R-esponse of BP E-lectrolytes T-ake Pulses I-schemic Episodes (TIA) C-omplications: 4C's
4 C's of Hypertension (Complications)	C- Coronary Artery Disease C- Coronary Rheumatic Fever C- Congestive Heart Failure C- Cardio Vascular Accident
Complications of Trauma Client (TRAUMATIC)	T-issue Perfusion Problems R-espiratory Problems A-nxiety U-nstable Clotting Factors M-alnutrition A-ltered Body Image T-hromboembolism I-nfection C-oping Problems
Cyanotic Defects: 4 T's	T- Tetralogy of Fallot T- Truncus Arteriosus T- Transportation of the Great Vessels T- Tricuspid Atresia
Cranial Nerve Mnemonic 01	OLympic (Olfactory) OPium (Optic) OCcupies (Oculomotor) TROubled (Trochlear) TRIathletes (Trigeminal) After (Abducens) Finishing (Facial) VEgas (Vestibulocochlear) Gambling (Glossopharyngeal) VAcations (Vagus) Still (Spinal Accessory) High (Hypoglossal)
Cranial Nerve Mnemonic 02	O- Oh O- Oh O- Oh T- To T- Touch A- And F - Feel A G - irl's V - agina S - So H- Heavenly
Cranial Nerve Mnemonic 03	O- On O -Old O- Obando T- Tower T- Top A- F- Filipino A - Army G - Guards V - Villages A - And H - Huts
Cranial Nerve Mnemonics (Sensory, Motor or Both)	S - Some S - Says M- Marilyn M- Monroe B - But M- My B- Brother S- Says B- Bridget B - Bardot M- Mmm M- Mmm
Cranial Nerve Mnemonics 02 (Sensory, Motor or Both)	S- Some S- Say M - Marry M- Money B- But M- My B - Brother S- Says B- Bad B- Business M - Marry M - Money
Nursing Care for Sprains and Strains (RICE)	R- Rest I - Ice C - Compression E- Elevation

Care of Client in Traction (TRACTION)	T- Temperature (Extremity, Infection) R - Ropes hang freely A - Alignment C - Circulation Check (5 P's) T- Type & Location of fracture I - Increase fluide Intake O - Overhead trapeze N - No weights on bed or floor
OB Non-Stress Test (NNN) 3 negatives in a row to interpret results of Non-Stress Test	N - Non-reactive N - Non- Stress is N - Not good
Severe Pre-Eclampsia (HELLP)	H- emolysis E- levated L- iver function tests L- ow P- latelet count
Assessment Tests for Fetal Well-Being (ALONE)	A- Amniocentesis L- L/S Ratio O - Oxytocin Test N - Non-Stress Test E - Estriol Level
Evalution of Episiotomy Healing (REEDA)	R- Redness E- Edema E - Ecchymosis D - Discharge, Drainage A - Approximation
Evalution of Episiotomy Healing (REEDA)	R- Redness E- Edema E - Ecchymosis D - Discharge, Drainage A - Approximation
Post-Partum Assessment (BUBBLE)	B-reasts U-terus B-owels B-ladder L-ochia E-pisiotomy/lateration/C-section incision
Tracheal Esophageal Fistula (3 C's)	C- Choking C- Coughing C - Cyanosis
Cleft Lip - Post Op Care (CLEFT LIP)	C-hoking L-ie on back E-valuate Airway F-eed Slowly T-eaching L-arger nipple opening I-ncidence incerase in males P-revent crust formation and aspiration
ADLs (Activity of Daily Living) BATTED	B-athing A-mbulation T-oileting T-ransfers E-ating D-ressing
IADLS (Instrumental Activities of Daily Living) SCUM	S-hopping C-ooking and Cleaning U-sing telephone or transportaiton M-anaging money and medications
Bleeding Precautions (RANDI)	R- Razor Electric/ Blades A- Aspirin N- No needles (esp. in small gauge) D- Do decrease in needle sticks) I - Injury (Protect from)
Canes and Walkers (COAL)	C- Cane O- Opposite A- Affected L- Leg
Canes and Walkers (WWAL) Wandering Wilma's Always Late	W- Walker W- With A- Affected L - Leg
Common Causes of Transient Incontinence (DIAPPERS)	D-elirium I-nfection A-trophic Urethra P-harmaceuticals P-sychologic E-xcess Urine Output R-estricted Mobility S-tool Impaction
Promotion of Normal Elimination (POOPER SCOOP)	P-osition O-utput O-ffer Fluids P-rivacy E-xercise R-eport Results S-ize (Amount) C-onsistency O-ccult Blood O-dor P-eristalsis
Emergency Trauma Assessment (ABCDEFGHI)	A-irway B-reathing C-irculation D-isability E-xamine F-ahrenheit G-et Vitals H-ead to Toe Assessment I-ntervention
Trauma Surgery (AMPLE) after initial assessment	A-llergies M-edications P-ast Medical History L-ast Meal E-vents Surrounding Injury
Trauma Surgery (AMPLE) after initial assessment	A-llergies M-edications P-ast Medical History L-ast Meal E-vents Surrounding Injury
6 P's of Dyspnea	P- Pulmonary Bronchial Constriction P- Possible Foreign Body P- Pulmonary Embolus P- Pneumothorax P- Pump Failure P- Pneumonia
Lidocaine Toxicity (SAMS)	S-lurred Speech A-ltered Central Nervous System M-uscle Twitching S-eizures
Lidocaine Toxicity (SAMS)	S-lurred Speech A-ltered Central Nervous System M-uscle Twitching S-eizures
TDCI (These Drugs Can	T - Theophyline D - Dilantin C - Coumadin I - Iosone (Erythromycin)

Interact)	
Serious Complications of Oral Birth Control Pills (ACHES)	A- Abdominal Pain C - Chest Pain H - Headache E - Eye Problems S - Severe Leg Pain
Emergency Drugs to LEAN on	L- Lidocaine E - Epinephrine A- Atropine Sulfate N - Narcan
Drugs for Bradycardia & low BP (IDEA)	I - Isoproterenol D - Dopamine E - Epinephrine A - Atropine Sulfate
Cholinergic Crisis (SLUD)	S-alivation L-acrimation U-rination D-efecation
Depression Assessment (SIG)	S-leep Disturbances I-nterest Decreased G-uilty Feelings
Energy Decreased (CAPS)	C-oncentration decreased A-ppetite P-sychomotor function decreased S-uicidal Ideations
5 A's to Alzheimer Diagnosis	A-mnesia A-nomia A-praxia A-gnosia A-phasia
Major Symptoms of a Manic Attack (DIG FAST)	D- Distractibility I - Indiscretion G - Grandiosity F- Flight of Ideas A- Activity Increase S- Sleep Deficit T - Talkative
3 P's of Blindness	P- Preventable P- Painless P- Permanent
Symptoms of Leukemia (ANT)	A- Anemia N- Neutropenia T- Thrombocytopenia
Exercise Guide for Diabetic Fitness (FIT)	F - Frequency (3x per week) I - Intensity (60-80% of Maximal Heart Rate) T- Time (Aerobic Activity)
Symptoms of Hypoxia (RAT BED)	Early Hypoxia: R-estlessness A-nxiety T-achycardia/ Tachypnea Late Hypoxia: B-radycardia E-xtreme Restlessness D-yspnea
Symptoms of Hypoxia (in Pediatrics) - FINES	F-eeding difficulty I-nspiratory Stridor N-ares Flares E-xpiratory Grunting S-ternal Retractions
Management of ASTHMA	A-drenergics (Albuterol) S-teroids T-heophylline H-ydration (IV) M-ask (Oxygen) A-ntibiotics
Epiglottitis (AIR RAID)	A-irway Closed I-ncreased Pulse R-estlessness R-etractions A-nxiety Increased I-nspiratory Stridor D-rooling
Blood Flow Through the Cardiac Valves (Tissue Paper My Assets)	T-ricuspid P-ulmonic M-itrial A-ortic
Immediate Treatment of a Myocardial Infarction Client (MONA)	M- Morphine O- Oxygen N- Nitroglycerine A- ASA
Treating CHF (UNLOAD FAST)	U-pright Position N-itrates (in low dose) L-asix O-xygen A-minophylline D-igoxin F-luids (decrease) A-fterload (decrease) S-odium restriction T-est (Dig level, ABGs, K level)
DEMENTIA	Make sure they don't have problems with: D-rug and alcohol E-yes and ears M-etabolic and endocrine disorders E-motional disorders N-eurologic disorders T-umors and trauma I-nfection A-rteriovascular disease
Osteoporosis Risk Factors (ACCESS)	A-lcohol Use C-orticosteroid Use C-alcium low E-strogen low S-moking S-edentary lifestyle/s ACCESS leads to OSTEOPOROSIS
Who needs dialysis? (Check the vowels: AEIOU)	A- Acid-Base Problems E- Electrolyte Problems I- Intoxications O- Overload of fluids U - Uremic Symptoms
Prostate Problems are no... FUN	F- Frequency U- Urgency N- Nocturia
BRAT Diet (for severe dehydration)	B- Banana R- Rice A- Apple T- Toasted Bread
Gluten Free Diet (ROW)	R- Rye O- Oats W- Wheat
Assess Changes in Senile	J- Judgment A- Affect M- Memory C- Cognition O- Orientation

Dementia (JAMCO)	
3 P's of Diabetes Mellitus - Type 1 Signs & Symptoms	P- Polyuria (excessive urination) P- Polydypsia (excessive thirst) P- Polyphagia (excessive hunger)
Right-Sided Heart Failure (HEAD)	H- Hepatomegaly E- Edema (Bipedal) A- Ascites D- Distended Neck Vein
Left-Sided Heart Failure (CHOP)	C- Cough H- Hemoptysis O- Orthopnea P- Pulmonary Congestion (crackles/rales)
Hyperkalemia Management (KIND)	K- Kayexalate (orally/ enema) I- Insulin N- Na HCO3 D- Diuretics (Furosemide & Thiazides)
Management of Myocardial Infarction (MONATAS)	M- Morphine O- Oxygen N- Nitrates (Nitroglycerin) A- Aspirin (ASA) T- Thormbolytics A- Anti-Coagulants S- Stool Softeners
Electrolytes - PISO	P- Potassium I- Inside S- Sodium O- Outside
Eating Disorder: ANOREXIA	Amenorrhea delayed No organic factors accounts for weight loss Obviously thin but feels FAT Refusal to maintain normal body weight Epigastric discomfort is common Xsymptoms (peculiar symptoms) Intense fears of gaining weight Always thinking of foods
Eating Disorder: BULIMIA	B-inge eating U-nder strict dieting L-acks control over-eating I-nduced vomiting M-inimum of to binge eating episodes I-ncrease/Persistent concern of body size/shape A-buse of diuretics & laxatives
Findings of a Bulimia client: WASHED	W-eight loss of 15% of original body weight A-menorrhea S-ocial withdrawal H-istory of high activity & achievement E-lectrolyte Imbalance D-epression/ Distorted Body Image
Outcome of Alcoholism: BAD	B- Brain Damage A- Alcoholic Hallucinosis D- Death
5 D's of Behavioral Problems of Alcoholism	D- Denial D- Dependency D- Demanding D- Destructive D- Domineering
Situations requiring Crisis Situation: RAPE	R- Ruthless A- Abusive P- Personal E- Experience
Warning Signs of a Child Abuse/ Neglect: CHILD ABUSE	Child's excessive knowledge on sex & abusive words Hair growth in various lengths Inconsistent stories from the child & parent/s Low self-esteem Depression Apathy, no emotion Bruised Unusual injuries Serious injuries Evidence of old injuries not reported
MI management: MONA	Morphine O2 Nitroglycerine Aspirin
HYPOGLYCEMIA: TIRED	T Tired I Irritability R Restless E Excessive hunger D Diaphoresis-Depression
HEART MURMURS: SPASM	S Stenosis P Partial obstruction A Aneurysms S Septal defect M Mitral regurgitation
Hyperthyroidism (s/s) : THYROIDISM	Tremor Heart rate up Yawning (fatigueability) Restlessness Oligomenorrhea & amenorrhea Intolerance to heat Diarrhea Irritability Sweating Muscle wasting & weight loss
PUPIL SIZE miotic & mydriatic	Miotic: Little word=Little pupil Mydriatic: Big word=Big pupil
Anticholingergics Side Effects: 4-CAN'Ts	Can't see Can't pee Can't spit Can't sh*t
5W's of common causes of post-op fever	Wind (think pneumonia, splinting, incentive spirometer exercises not done, DB+ coughing not done) Water (dehydration...) Wound (infection, dehiscence...) Walking (PE...) Wonder drug (approriate antibiotic...)
Acute Pancreatitis: I GET SMASHED	Idiopathic Gallstone E - EtOH Trauma Steroids Mumps (paramyxovirus) and other viruses (EBV, CMV) Autoimmune Scorpion sting / snake bite H ypercalcemia, hyperlipidemia and hypothermia E - ERCP Drugs, duodenal ulcers
To apply a telemetry	White over right (top right shoulder) Black beside the white (Over lt

monitor:	shoulder) Checkers (red below the black) Christmas (Green beside the red) Then ofcourse, the brown will be in the middle!
The HYPERKALEMIA "Machine" - Causes of Increased Serum K+	M - Medications - ACE inhibitors, NSAIDS A - Acidosis - Metabolic and respiratory C - Cellular destruction - Burns, traumatic injury H - Hypoaldosteronism, hemolysis I - Intake - Excesssive N - Nephrons, renal failure E - Excretion - Impaired
Signs and Symptoms of Increased Serum K+: MURDER	M - Muscle weakness U - Urine, oliguria, anuria R- Respiratory distress D - Decreased cardiac contractility E - ECG changes R - Reflexes, hyperreflexia, or areflexia (flaccid)
HYPERNATREMIA "You Are Fried"	F - Fever (low grade), flushed skin R - Restless (irritable) I - Increased fluid retention and increased BP E - Edema (peripheral and pitting) D - Decreased urinary output, dry mouth
"CATS" of "HYPOCALCEMIA"	C - Convulsions A- Arrhythmias T - Tetany S - Spasms and stridor
HYPERNATREMIA	SALT S = Skin flushed A = Agitation L = Low-grade fever T = Thirst

Mnemonics for NCLEX

Question	Answer
The 5 A's of Alzheimers	1. Amnesia (memory loss) 2. Anomia (unable to recall names of objects) 3. Apraxia (inability to perform particular purposive actions) 4. Agonsia (inability to interpret sensations & recognize things) 5. Aphasia (inability to understand/express speech)
Bipolar Mania Symptoms	D.I.G. F.A.S.T. Distractibility Indiscretion Grandiosity Flight of Ideas Activity Increase Sleep Deficit Talkative
Risk factors for primary hypertension: SOSAD IC	SOSAD IC •Sodium and fat intake •Obesity •Stress •Alcohol •D vitamin deficiency •Inactivity •Caffeine
Endocarditis signs FROM JANE	FROM JANE • Fever • Roth's spots • Osler's nodes • Murmur • Janeway lesions • Anemia • Nail hemorrhage (splinter hemorrhages) • Emboli
Shock—Stages "CPR"	"CPR" • Compensatory Stage • Progressive Stage • Refractory Stage
Shock—Causes "HAVANA"	"HAVANA" • Hypovolemia • Adrenal Crisis • Vascular Stasis • Acute Respiratory Obstruction • Neurogenic • Anaphylaxis
Hypertension—Causes Use the ABCDE method to identify secondary causes.	ABCDE secondary causes • Aldosterone/Apnea • Bad kidney/Bruits • Catecholamines/Cushings syndrome • Drugs/Diet • Endocrine
Oxygen Dissociation—Right Shift A right shift is a DATE with CO2	A right shift is a DATE with CO2 • 2,3 Diphosphoglycerate DPG • Acidosis • Temperature • Exercise
Acid-Base Balance ROME	ROME Respiratory Opposite • pH up PCO2 down = Alkalosis • pH down PCO2 up = Acidosis Metabolic Equal • pH up HCO3 up = Alkalosis • pH down HCO3 down = Acidosis
RUB MUB Compensation	Respiratory Uses Bicarb, Metabolic Uses Breathing • Respiratory Acidosis, Retain Bicarb • Respiratory Alkalosis, Excrete Bicarb • Metabolic Acidosis, Increase Breathing • Metabolic Alkalosis, Decrease Breathing
Dyspnea—Signs 6 Ps	6 Ps •Pneumonia •Pulmonary Bronchial Constriction •Possible Foreign Body •Pulmonary Embolus •Pneumothorax •Pump Failure
Hypoxia Symptoms: RAT BED	RAT BED • Early Hypoxia: Restlessness Anxiety Tachycardia/Tachypnea • Late Hypoxia: Bradycardia Extreme Restlessness Dyspnea
Asthma Management ASTHMA:	ASTHMA: •Adrenergics (Albuterol) •Steroids •Theophylline •Hydration (IV) •Mask (Oxygen) •Antibiotics (Infection)
Cranial nerves order "Oh, oh, oh, to touch and feel a girl's vagina. Such heaven!"	CN I: olfactory CN II: optic CN III: oculomotor CN IV: trochlear CN V: trigeminal CN VI: abducens CN VII: facial CN VIII: auditory or vestibulocochlear CN IX: glossopharyngeal CN X: vagus CN XI: spinal accessory CN XII: hypoglossal
Cranial nerves : S: sensory; m: motor; b: both "Some say marry money but my brother says big brains matter more"	S- I: olfactory S- II: optic M- III: oculomotor M- IV: trochlear B- V: trigeminal M- VI: abducens B- VII: facial S- VIII: auditory or vestibulocochlear B- IX: glossopharyngeal B- X: vagus M- XI: spinal accessory M- XII: hypoglossal
Hypothalamus Functions Hypothalamus wears TAN HATS	Hypothalamus wears TAN HATS • Thirst and water balance • Adenohypophysis • Neurohypophysis • Hunger and satiety • Autonomic regulation • Temperature regulation • Sexual urges and emotions
Blood Glucose—Hormonal Influence Hormones that Increase Blood Glucose	Hormones that Increase Blood Glucose "STENGG" • Somatotropin (growth hormone) • Thyroid hormones (thyroxine

"STENGG"	and triiodothyronine) • Epinephrine • Norepinephrine • Glucagon • Glucocorticosteroids
Insulin Functions on Cells INsulIN stimulates 2 things to go IN 2 cells:	INsulIN stimulates 2 things to go IN 2 cells: Potassium and Glucose.
Hypoglycemia TIRED	TIRED • Tachycardia • Irritability • Restlessness • Excessive Hunger • Diaphoresis Rhyme Cold and clammy, need some candy
Hyperglycemia 3 P's	3 P's • Polyphagia • Polydipsia • Polyuria Rhyme Hot and dry, sugar high
Hisutism—The 5 Hs 5 Hs	5 Hs • Hirsutism • Hyperplasia of gums • Harm to kidneys • Hypertension • Hyperglycemia
Attenuated (live/weakened) Vaccines "ROME Is My Best Place To Yell!"	"ROME Is My Best Place To Yell!" • Rubella • Oral polio vaccine • Measles • Epidemic typhus • Influenza • Mumps • BCG • Plague • Typhoid oral vaccine • Yellow fever
White Blood Cells (In order of decreasing numbers.) "Nobody Likes My Educational Background" or "Never Let Monkeys Eat Bananas"	•Neutrophils •Lymphocytes •Monocytes •Eosinophils •Basophils
Multiple Myeloma Symptoms CRAB:	CRAB: • Calcium level elevated • Renal failure • Anemia • Bone breakdown and resorption
AIDS—The Cells Attacked	AIDS—The Cells Attacked AIDS is 4 letters long. AIDS attacks CD4 T cells.
Cancer's Early Warning Signs CAUTION UP	•Change bowel/bladder •A lesion doesnt heal •Unusual bleeding/discharge •Thickening/lump breast/elsewhere •Indigestion/difficulty swallowing •Obvious change wart/mole •Nagging cough/persistent hoarseness •Unexplained weight loss •Pernicious Anemia
Burns—Rule of Nines and Rule of Palms Total body surface area (TBSA): Rule of Nines:	• 9% Head • 9% Chest • 9% Abdomen • 9% Upper back • 9% Lower back • 9% Anterior leg, each • 9% Posterior leg, each • 9% Entire arm, each • 1% Genitalia/perineum Rule of Palms: • 1% Palm of hand
Melanoma Characteristics ABCDE	ABCDE • Asymmetrical • Borders irregular • Color dark and variation • Diameter is large (> 6MM) • Evolving
Scleroderma CREST syndrome:	CREST syndrome: • Calcinosis • Raynaud's Syndrome • Esophageal Motility Disorder • Sclerodactyly • Telangiectasia
Syphilis—Primary PRESS	PRESS • Painless lesion • Regional lymphadenopathy • Exudate • Single lesion • Sexual contact can cause
Syphilis—Secondary CAMP	CAMP • Condyloma lata • Acute Infection symptoms (fever, sore throat, malaise, weight loss) • Mucocutaneous lesion, mucous patches • Papules & Pustules
Syphilis—Tertiary CLASS	CLASS • Cardiovascular disorder • Late benign syphilis (gumma) • Asymptomatic Neurosyphilis • Symptomatic Neurosyphilis • Seizures and apathy (signs of meningeal involvement)
Sprains and Strains—Interventions RICE	RICE • Rest • Ice • Compression • Elevation
Traction Care TRACTION	TRACTION • Temperature (Extremity, Infection) • hang freely • Alignment • Circulation Check (5 P's) • Type & Location of fracture • Increase fluide intake • Overhead trapeze • No weights on bed or floor
Canes and Walkers COAL and WWAL	COAL • Cane • Opposite • Affected • Leg WWAL • Walker • With • Affected • Leg
Autonomic Nervous System Functions Rhyme	Sympathetic: fight or flight Parasympathetic: rest and digest
Prioritization The order in which we use the strategies in a priority question: PHAN	PHAN •Priority •Hierarchy •ABCs •Nursing Process

Nursing Process How to find the correct answer by using the nursing process. Assess before you implement! ADPIE:	Assess before you implement! ADPIE: •Assessment •Diagnosis •Planning •Implementation •Evaluation
Patient Handoff Report I-SBAR patient handoff reporting supports the National Patient Safety Goal #2, "to improve effectiveness of communication among caregivers."	I-SBAR: •Identify •Situation •Background •Assessment •Recommendation
Inflammation—Signs PRISH	PRISH • Pain • Redness • Immobility (loss of function) • Swelling • Heat
Activities of Daily Living (ADL) BATTED	BATTED •Bathing •Ambulation •Toileting •Transfers •Eating •Dressing
Instrumental Activities of Daily Living (IADL) SCUM	SCUM •Shopping •Cooking and Cleaning •Using telephone or transportation •Managing money and medications
Oxygen Dissociation—Right Shift A right shift is a DATE with CO2	A right shift is a DATE with CO2 •2,3 Diphosphoglycerate DPG •Acidosis •Temperature •Exercise
Gestation—Bartholomew's Rule of Fours	Gestation—Bartholomew's Rule of Fours • 12 Weeks: Symphisis pubis • 16 weeks: Midway between symphysis pubis and umbilicus • 20 weeks: Umbilicus • 36 weeks: Xiphoid process
Teratogens TAP CAP	TAP CAP • Thalidomide • Alcohol • Progestins • Corticosteroids • Aspirin • Phenytoin
Clubfoot—Deformities InAdEquate	InAdEquate • Inversion • Adduction • Equinus
Esophageal Atresia and Tracheoesophageal Fistula 3 C's	3 C's • Coughing • Choking • Cyanosis
Nephritic Syndrome PHARAOH	PHARAOH • Proteinuria & Edema • Hematuria • Azotemia • RBC casts • Anti-strep titres (If post-strep) • Oliguria • Hypertension
Kidney Layers "Our Careers In Medicine"	Kidney layers "Our Careers In Medicine" • Outer cortex • Inner medulla
Flow of fluid through the Kidney "Be Prepared To Look Happy During Computer-based Testing"	Flow of fluid "Be Prepared To Look Happy During Computer-based Testing" •Bowmans capsule •Proximal Tubules •Loop Henle •Distal and Convoluted Tubules
Liver Functions PUSH DoG	PUSH DoG • Protein synthesis • Ureas synthesis • Storage • Hormone synthesis • Detoxification • Glucose and fat metabolism
Nephrotic Syndrome People Have Endless Appetites	People Have Endless Appetites • Proteinuria • Hyperlipidemia • Edema • Albuminuria & hypoalbuminemia
Intestinal Components Bowel Components (in order): Dow Jones Industrial Can't Choose Stocks	Dow Jones Industrial Can't Choose Stocks • Duodenum • Jejunum • Ileum • Cecum • Colon • Sigmoid
Streptococcus pyogenes—Diseases GET NIPPLES	GET NIPPLES • Glomerulonephritis • Endocarditis (Heart Valves) • Toxic shock syndrome • Necrotizing fasciitis and myositis • Impetigo • Pharyngitis • Pneumonia • Lymphangitis • Erysipelas and cellulitis • Scarlet fever/Rheumatic Fever
Common Cold—Causes CREAR:	CREAR: • Coronavirus • Rhinoviruses • Enterovirus • Adenovirus • Respiratory Syncytial Virus (RSV)
Rubella, Congenital—Signs "Rubber Ducky, I so Blue"	"Rubber Ducky, I so Blue" • Rubella • Patent ductus arteriosus • Eyes • Blueberry muffin rash
Staph aureus caused by SOFT PAINS	Staph aureus caused by SOFT PAINS • Skin infections • Osteomyelitis • Food poisoning • Toxic shock syndrome • Pneumonia • Acute endocarditis • Infective arthritis • Necrotizing fasciitis • Sepsis
E. coli causes DUNG	E. coli causes DUNG • Diarrhea • UTI • Neonatal meningitis • Gram negative sepsis

Pseudomonas Aeruginosa P-S-E-U & A-E-R-U-G-I-N-O-S-A	P-S-E-U •Pneumonia •Sepsis •External otits media •UTI A-F-R-U-G-I-N-O-S-A •Aerobic •Exotoxin A •Rod •UTI, burns&infection •Green blue pigment •Iron containing lesions •Neg. gram,non lactose fermenting •Oxidase pos. •Sepsis •Adherence pili
Triage color system Red, Yellow, Green, Black 32 can do	Red–Don't with within 15 mins they will die, ABC problem, above 30, no pulse, mentally confused Yellow–30 mins, not ABC but still wounded, above 30, pulse, mental status normal Green–emotional issues, walking wounded Black-dead, less 30 RR
heat vs cold first	Use heat first for muscles Use cold first for nerves
Walking Up and Down stairs with crutches	Good people go to heaven (good leg up) Bad people go to hell (bad leg down)
Naegele's rule	1st day of LMP - 3 months (don't forget to adjust year if needed) + 7 days (don't forget to adjust the month if needed)
Stages of Labor	1. Getting ready to Push a. Latent – 0-3, little to no pain b. Active – 3-7, c. Transition – 7-10, effacement 100% 2. Pushing = Baby 3. Placenta 4. Bonding
Postpartum Lochia changes	Rubra (3-5 days, blood & clots) Serosa (10 days, pink) Alba (up to 2-5 weeks, Should not be longer than 6 weeks, white/creamy)
Decels and Accels (FHR) Change> Cause> What to do VEAL >CHOP> MINE	Variable Dec>Cord compression>Move(Trendelenburg>Csection) Early Dec>Head Compression>Identify Labor(active good, no progression bad) Accel>OK>Nothing Late Dec>Placenta Insufficiency>Execute actions NOW (move, turn off Pitocin, ^fluids, O2, Csection)
PROM vs. PPROM	*PROM(Premature Rupture of Membrane) = More than 1 hour before onset of labor, Use Pitocin to get things moving *PPROM (Preterm)= 37 weeks and More than 1 hour before onset of labor, Risk for infection (prophylactic ATB), Bed Rest, Steroids (if needed)
Parkland Formula (Fluid Replacement) for Burns	[4 x wgt (kg) x TBSA %] / 2 = ANSWER ANSWER – give in first 8 hours ANSWER – give in next 16 hours

Mnemonics
Flash Cards
Questions on ODD pages and Answers on EVEN pages

Steps in the Nursing Process ADPIE (A Delicious PIE)	Steps in the Nursing Process AAPIE (An Apple Pie)
Acid-Base (ROME)	Inflammation (HIPER)

<table>
<tr>
<td>A-ssessment A-nanlysis P-lanning I-mplementation E-valuation</td>
<td>A-ssessment D- iagnosis P-lanning I-mplementation E-valuaton</td>
</tr>
<tr>
<td>H-eat I-nduration P-ain E-dema R-edness</td>
<td>R-espiratory O-pposite M-etabolic E-qual</td>
</tr>
</table>

CANCER'S Early Warning Signs CAUTION UP	CANCER Interventions
Adrenal Gland Hormones (SSS)	Hypoglycemia (TIRED) - an abnormal decrease of blood in the sugar

C-omfort A-ltered Body Image N-utrition C-hemotherapy E-valuate response to meds R-espite for caretakers	Change in bowel/bladder A lesion doesn't heal Unusual bleeding/discharge Thickening lump in breast/elsewhere Indigestion/difficulty swallowing Obvious changes wart/mole Nagging cough/persistent hoarseness Unexplained weight loss
T-achycardia I-rritability R-estless E-xcessive Hunger D-iaphoresis/ Depression	S-ugar (Glucocorticoids) S-alt (Mineralcorticoids) S-ex (Androgens)

<table>
<tr><td>Pulmonary Edema (MAD DOG)</td><td>5 P's of Circulatory Checks</td></tr>
<tr><td>4 C's of Hypertension (Complications)</td><td>Hypertension Nursing Care (DIURETIC)</td></tr>
</table>

P-Pain P-Paresthesia P-Paralysis P-Pulse P-Pallor (Paleness)	M-Morphine A-Aminophylline D- Digitalis D-Diuretics (Lasix) O- Oxygen G- ases (Blood Gases ABG's)
D-aily Weight I- ntake and Output (I & O) U- rine Output R-esponse of BP E-lectrolytes T-ake Pulses I-schemic Episodes (TIA) C-omplications: 4C's	C- Coronary Artery Disease C-Coronary Rheumatic Fever C-Congestive Heart Failure C-Cardio Vascular Accident

Complications of Trauma Client (TRAUMATIC)	Cyanotic Defects: 4 T's
Cranial Nerve Mnemonic 02	Cranial Nerve Mnemonic 01

T- Tetralogy of Fallot T- Truncus Arteriosus T- Transportation of the Great Vessels T- Tricuspid Atresia	T-issue Perfusion Problems R-espiratory Problems A-nxiety U-nstable Clotting Factors M-alnutrition A-ltered Body Image T-hromboembolism I-nfection C-oping Problems
OLympic (Olfactory) OPium (Optic) OCcupies (Oculomotor) TROubled (Trochlear) TRIathletes (Trigeminal) After (Abducens) Finishing (Facial) VEgas (Vestibulocochlear) Gambling (Glossopharyngeal) VAcations (Vagus) Still (Spinal	O- Oh O- Oh O- Oh T- To T-Touch A- And F - Feel A G - irl's V - agina S - So H-Heavenly

<table>
<tr><td>Cranial Nerve Mnemonic 03</td><td>Cranial Nerve Mnemonics
(Sensory, Motor or Both)</td></tr>
<tr><td>Nursing Care for Sprains and
Strains (RICE)</td><td>Cranial Nerve Mnemonics 02
(Sensory, Motor or Both)</td></tr>
</table>

S - Some S - Says M- Marilyn M- Monroe B - But M- My B- Brother S- Says B- Bridget B - Bardot M- Mmm M- Mmm	O- On O -Old O- Obando T- Tower T- Top A- F- Filipino A - Army G - Guards V - Villages A - And H - Huts
S- Some S- Say M - Marry M- Money B- But M- My B - Brother S- Says B- Bad B- Business M - Marry M - Money	R- Rest I - Ice C - Compression E- Elevation

Care of Client in Traction (TRACTION)	OB Non-Stress Test (NNN) 3 negatives in a row to interpret results of Non-Stress Test
Assessment Tests for Fetal Well-Being (ALONE)	Severe Pre-Eclampsia (HELLP)

N - Non-reactive N - Non-Stress is N - Not good	T- Temperature (Extremity, Infection) R - Ropes hang freely A - Alignment C - Circulation Check (5 P's) T- Type & Location of fracture I - Increase fluide intake O - Overhead trapeze N - No weights on bed or floor
H- emolysis E- levated L- iver function tests L- ow P- latelet count	A- Amniocentesis L- L/S Ratio O - Oxytocin Test N - Non-Stress Test E - Estriol Level

Evalution of Episiotomy Healing (REEDA)	Evalution of Episiotomy Healing (REEDA)
Tracheal Esophageal Fistula (3 C's)	Post-Partum Assessment (BUBBLE)

R- Redness E- Edema E - Ecchymosis D - Discharge, Drainage A - Approximation	R- Redness E- Edema E - Ecchymosis D - Discharge, Drainage A - Approximation
B-reasts U-terus B-owels B-ladder L-ochia E-pisiotomy/lateration/C-section incision	C- Choking C- Coughing C - Cyanosis

Cleft Lip - Post Op Care (CLEFT LIP)	ADLs (Activity of Daily Living) BATTED
Bleeding Precautions (RANDI)	IADLS (Instrumental Activities of Daily Living) SCUM

B-athing A-mbulation T-oileting T-ransfers E-ating D-ressing	C-hoking L-ie on back E-valuate Airway F-eed Slowly T-eaching L-arger nipple opening I-ncidence incerase in males P-revent crust formation and aspiration
S-hopping C-ooking and Cleaning U-sing telephone or transportaiton M-anaging money and medications	R- Razor Electric/ Blades A- Aspirin N- No needles (esp. in small gauge) D- Do decrease in needle sticks) I - Injury (Protect from)

<table>
<tr><td>

Canes and Walkers (COAL)

</td><td>

Canes and Walkers (WWAL)
Wandering Wilma's Always
Late

</td></tr>
<tr><td>

Promotion of Normal
Elimination (POOPER
SCOOP)

</td><td>

Common Causes of Transient
Incontinence (DIAPPERS)

</td></tr>
</table>

W- Walker W- With A-Affected L - Leg	C- Cane O- Opposite A-Affected L- Leg
D-elirium I-nfection A-trophic Urethra P-harmaceuticals P-sychologic E-xcess Urine Output R-estricted Mobility S-tool Impaction	P-osition O-utput O-ffer Fluids P-rivacy E-xercise R-eport Results S-ize (Amount) C-onsistency O-ccult Blood O-dor P-eristalsis

<table>
<tr><td>Emergency Trauma Assessment (ABCDEFGHI)</td><td>Trauma Surgery (AMPLE) after initial assessment</td></tr>
<tr><td>6 P's of Dyspnea</td><td>Trauma Surgery (AMPLE) after initial assessment</td></tr>
</table>

A-llergies M-edications P-ast Medical History L-ast Meal E-vents Surrounding Injury	A-irway B-reathing C-irculation D-isability E-xamine F-ahrenheit G-et Vitals H-ead to Toe Assessment I-ntervention
A-llergies M-edications P-ast Medical History L-ast Meal E-vents Surrounding Injury	P- Pulmonary Bronchial Constriction P- Possible Foreign Body P- Pulmonary Embolus P- Pneumothorax P- Pump Failure P- Pneumonia

<table>
<tr><td>Lidocaine Toxicity (SAMS)</td><td>Lidocaine Toxicity (SAMS)</td></tr>
<tr><td>Serious Complications of Oral Birth Control Pills (ACHES)</td><td>TDCI (These Drugs Can Interact)</td></tr>
</table>

S-lurred Speech A-ltered Central Nervous System M-uscle Twitching S-eizures	S-lurred Speech A-ltered Central Nervous System M-uscle Twitching S-eizures
T - Theophyline D - Dilantin C - Coumadin I - Iosone (Erythromycin)	A- Abdominal Pain C - Chest Pain H - Headache E - Eye Problems S - Severe Leg Pain

Emergency Drugs to LEAN on	Drugs for Bradycardia & low BP (IDEA)
Depression Assessment (SIG)	Cholinergic Crisis (SLUD)

I - Isoproterenol D - Dopamine E - Epinephrine A - Atropine Sulfate	L- Lidocaine E - Epinephrine A- Atropine Sulfate N - Narcan
S-alivation L-acrimation U-rination D-efecation	S-leep Disturbances I-nterest Decreased G-uilty Feelings

<table>
<tr><td>Energy Decreased (CAPS)</td><td>5 A's to Alzheimer Diagnosis</td></tr>
<tr><td>3 P's of Blindness</td><td>Major Symptoms of a Manic Attack (DIG FAST)</td></tr>
</table>

A-mnesia A-nomia A-praxia A-gnosia A-phasia	C-oncentration decreased A-ppetite P-sychomotor function decreased S-uicidal Ideations
D- Distractibility I - Indiscretion G - Grandiosity F- Flight of Ideas A- Activity Increase S- Sleep Deficit T - Talkative	P- Preventable P- Painless P- Permanent

<table>
<tr><td>Symptoms of Leukemia (ANT)</td><td>Exercise Guide for Diabetic Fitness (FIT)</td></tr>
<tr><td>Symptoms of Hypoxia (in Pediatrics) - FINES</td><td>Symptoms of Hypoxia (RAT BED)</td></tr>
</table>

F - Frequency (3x per week) I - Intensity (60-80% of Maximal Heart Rate) T- Time (Aerobic Activity)	A- Anemia N- Neutropenia T- Thrombocytopenia
Early Hypoxia: R-estlessness A-nxiety T-achycardia/ Tachypnea Late Hypoxia: B-radycardia E-xtreme Restlessness D-yspnea	F-eeding difficulty I-nspiratory Stridor N-ares Flares E-xpiratory Grunting S-ternal Retractions

Management of ASTHMA	Epiglottitis (AIR RAID)
Immediate Treatment of a Myocardial Infarction Client (MONA)	Blood Flow Through the Cardiac Valves (Tissue Paper My Assets)

A-irway Closed I-ncreased Pulse R-estlessness R-etractions A-nxiety Increased I-nspiratory Stridor D-rooling	A-drenergics (Albuterol) S-teroids T-heophylline H-ydration (IV) M-ask (Oxygen) A-ntibiotics
T-ricuspid P-ulmonic M-itrial A-ortic	M- Morphine O- Oxygen N- Nitroglycerine A- ASA

Treating CHF (UNLOAD FAST)	DEMENTIA
Who needs dialysis? (Check the vowels: AEIOU)	Osteoporosis Risk Factors (ACCESS)

Make sure they don't have problems with: D-rug and alcohol E-yes and ears M-etabolic and endocrine disorders E-motional disorders N-eurologic disorders T-umors and trauma I-nfection A-rteriovascular disease	U-pright Position N-itrates (in low dose) L-asix O-xygen A-minophylline D-igoxin F-luids (decrease) A-fterload (decrease) S-odium restriction T-est (Dig level, ABGs, K level)
A-lcohol Use C-orticosteroid Use C-alcium low E-strogen low S-moking S-edentary lifestyle/s ACCESS leads to OSTEOPOROSIS	A- Acid-Base Problems E-Electrolyte Problems I-Intoxications O- Overload of fluids U - Uremic Symptoms

<table>
<tr><td>Prostate Problems are no...
FUN</td><td>BRAT Diet (for severe dehydration)</td></tr>
<tr><td>Assess Changes in Senile Dementia (JAMCO)</td><td>Gluten Free Diet (ROW)</td></tr>
</table>

<table>
<tr><td>B- Banana R- Rice A- Apple T- Toasted Bread</td><td>F- Frequency U- Urgency N- Nocturia</td></tr>
<tr><td>R- Rye O- Oats W- Wheat</td><td>J- Judgment A- Affect M- Memory C- Cognition O- Orientation</td></tr>
</table>

3 P's of Diabetes Mellitus - Type 1 Signs & Symptoms	Right-Sided Heart Failure (HEAD)
Hyperkalemia Management (KIND)	Left-Sided Heart Failure (CHOP)

H- Hepatomegaly E- Edema (Bipedal) A- Ascites D- Distended Neck Vein	P- Polyuria (excessive urination) P- Polydypsia (excessive thirst) P- Polyphagia (excessive hunger)
C- Cough H- Hemoptysis O- Orthopnea P- Pulmonary Congestion (crackles/ rales)	K- Kayexalate (orally/ enema) I- Insulin N- Na HCO3 D- Diuretics (Furosemide & Thiazides)

Management of Myocardial Infarction (MONATAS)	Electrolytes - PISO
Eating Disorder: BULIMIA	Eating Disorder: ANOREXIA

P- Potassium I- Inside S- Sodium O- Outside	M- Morphine O- Oxygen N- Nitrates (Nitroglycerin) A- Aspirin (ASA) T- Thormbolytics A- Anti-Coagulants S- Stool Softeners
Amenorrhea delayed No organic factors accounts for weight loss Obviously thin but feels FAT Refusal to maintain normal body weight Epigastric discomfort is common Xsymptoms (peculiar symptoms) Intense fears of gaining weight Always	B-inge eating U-nder strict dieting L-acks control over-eating I-nduced vomiting M-inimum of to binge eating episodes I-ncrease/Persistent concern of body size/shape A-buse of diuretics & laxatives

Findings of a Bulimia client: WASHED	Outcome of Alcoholism: BAD
Situations requiring Crisis Situation: RAPE	5 D's of Behavioral Problems of Alcoholism

B- Brain Damage A- Alcoholic Hallucinosis D- Death	W-eight loss of 15% of original body weight A-menorrhea S-ocial withdrawal H-istory of high activity & achievement E-lectrolyte Imbalance D-epression/ Distorted Body Image
D- Denial D- Dependency D- Demanding D- Destructive D- Domineering	R- Ruthless A- Abusive P- Personal E- Experience

Warning Signs of a Child Abuse/ Neglect: CHILD ABUSE	MI management: MONA
HEART MURMURS: SPASM	HYPOGLYCEMIA: TIRED

Morphine O2 Nitroglycerine Aspirin	Child's excessive knowledge on sex & abusive words Hair growth in various lengths Inconsistent stories from the child & parent/s Low self-esteem Depression Apathy, no emotion Bruised Unusual injuries Serious injuries Evidence of old injuries not
T Tired I Irritability R Restless E Excessive hunger D Diaphoresis-Depression	S Stenosis P Partial obstruction A Aneurysms S Septal defect M Mitral regurgitation

<table>
<tr>
<td>Hyperthyroidism (s/s) :
THYROIDISM</td>
<td>PUPIL SIZE miotic &
mydriatic</td>
</tr>
<tr>
<td>5W's of common causes of
post-op fever</td>
<td>Anticholinergics Side Effects:
4-CAN'Ts</td>
</tr>
</table>

Miotic: Little word=Little pupil Mydriatic: Big word=Big pupil	Tremor Heart rate up Yawning (fatigueability) Restlessness Oligomenorrhea & amenorrhea Intolerance to heat Diarrhea Irritability Sweating Muscle wasting & weight loss
Can't see Can't pee Can't spit Can't sh*t	Wind (think pneumonia, splinting, incentive spirometer exercises not done, DB+ coughing not done) Water (dehydration...) Wound (infection, dehiscence...) Walking (PE...) Wonder drug (approriate antibiotic...)

Acute Pancreatitis: I GET SMASHED	To apply a telemetry monitor:
Signs and Symptoms of Increased Serum K+: MURDER	The HYPERKALEMIA "Machine" - Causes of Increased Serum K+

White over right (top right shoulder) Black beside the white (Over lt shoulder) Checkers (red below the black) Christmas (Green beside the red) Then ofcourse, the brown will be in the middle!	Idiopathic Gallstone E - EtOH Trauma Steroids Mumps (paramyxovirus) and other viruses (EBV, CMV) Autoimmune Scorpion sting / snake bite H ypercalcemia, hyperlipidemia and hypothermia E - ERCP Drugs, duodenal ulcers
M - Medications - ACE inhibitors, NSAIDS A - Acidosis - Metabolic and respiratory C - Cellular destruction - Burns, traumatic injury H - Hypoaldosteronism, hemolysis I - Intake - Excesssive N - Nephrons, renal failure E - Excretion - Impaired	M - Muscle weakness U - Urine, oliguria, anuria R- Respiratory distress D - Decreased cardiac contractility E - ECG changes R - Reflexes, hyperreflexia, or areflexia (flaccid)

<table>
<tr><td>HYPERNATREMIA "You Are Fried"</td><td>"CATS" of "HYPOCALCEMIA"</td></tr>
<tr><td></td><td>HYPERNATREMIA</td></tr>
</table>

C - ConvulsionsA-ArrhythmiasT - TetanyS - Spasms and stridor	F - Fever (low grade), flushed skin R - Restless (irritable) I - Increased fluid retention and increased BP E - Edema (peripheral and pitting) D - Decreased urinary output, dry mouth
SALTS = Skin flushedA = AgitationL = Low-grade feverT = Thirst	

| The 5 A's of Alzheimers | Bipolar Mania Symptoms |
| Endocarditis signs FROM JANE | Risk factors for primary hypertension: SOSAD IC |

D.I.G. F.A.S.T.	1. Amnesia (memory loss)
Distractibility Indiscretion Grandiosity Flight of Ideas	2. Anomia (unable to recall names of objects) 3. Apraxia (inability to perform particular purposive actions) 4. Agonsia (inability to interpret sensations & recognize things) 5. Aphasia (inability to
SOSAD IC •Sodium and fat intake •Obesity •Stress •Alcohol •D vitamin deficiency •Inactivity •Caffeine	**FROM JANE** • Fever • Roth's spots • Osler's nodes • Murmur • Janeway lesions • Anemia • Nail hemorrhage (splinter hemorrhages)

Shock—Stages "CPR"	Shock—Causes "HAVANA"
Oxygen Dissociation—Right Shift A right shift is a DATE with CO2	Hypertension—Causes Use the ABCDE method to identify secondary causes.

"HAVANA" • Hypovolemia • Adrenal Crisis • Vascular Stasis • Acute Respiratory Obstruction • Neurogenic • Anaphylaxis	**"CPR"** • Compensatory Stage • Progressive Stage • Refractory Stage
ABCDE secondary causes • Aldosterone/Apnea • Bad kidney/Bruits • Catecholamines/Cushings syndrome • Drugs/Diet • Endocrine	A right shift is a DATE with CO_2 • 2,3 Diphosphoglycerate DPG • Acidosis • Temperature • Exercise

<table>
<tr><td>Acid-Base Balance
ROME</td><td>RUB MUB Compensation</td></tr>
<tr><td>Hypoxia Symptoms: RAT
BED</td><td>Dyspnea—Signs
6 Ps</td></tr>
</table>

Respiratory Uses Bicarb, Metabolic Uses Breathing	ROME
Respiratory Uses Bicarb, Metabolic Uses Breathing • Respiratory Acidosis, Retain Bicarb • Respiratory Alkalosis, Excrete Bicarb • Metabolic Acidosis, Increase Breathing • Metabolic Alkalosis,	ROME Respiratory Opposite • pH up PCO2 down = Alkalosis • pH down PCO2 up = Acidosis Metabolic Equal • pH up HCO3 up = Alkalosis
6 Ps •Pneumonia •Pulmonary Bronchial Constriction •Possible Foreign Body •Pulmonary Embolus •Pneumothorax •Pump Failure	RAT BED • Early Hypoxia: Restlessness Anxiety Tachycardia/ Tachypnea • Late Hypoxia: Bradycardia Extreme Restlessness

<table>
<tr><td>

Asthma Management
ASTHMA:

</td><td>

Cranial nerves order
"Oh, oh, oh, to touch and feel a girl's vagina. Such heaven!"

</td></tr>
<tr><td>

Hypothalamus Functions
Hypothalamus wears TAN HATS

</td><td>

Cranial nerves : S: sensory; m: motor; b: both
"Some say marry money but my brother says big brains matter more"

</td></tr>
</table>

CN I: olfactory CN II: optic CN III: oculomotor CN IV: trochlear CN V: trigeminal CN VI: abducens CN VII: facial CN VIII: auditory or vestibulocochlear	ASTHMA: •Adrenergics (Albuterol) •Steroids •Theophylline •Hydration (IV) •Mask (Oxygen) •Antibiotics (Infection)
S- I: olfactory S- II: optic M- III: oculomotor M- IV: trochlear B- V: trigeminal M- VI: abducens B- VII: facial S- VIII: auditory or vestibulocochlear	Hypothalamus wears TAN HATS • Thirst and water balance • Adenohypophysis • Neurohypophysis • Hunger and satiety • Autonomic regulation • Temperature regulation

| Blood Glucose—Hormonal Influence
Hormones that Increase Blood Glucose "STENGG" | Insulin Functions on Cells
INsulIN stimulates 2 things to go IN 2 cells: |
| Hyperglycemia
3 P's | Hypoglycemia
TIRED |

INsulIN stimulates 2 things to go IN 2 cells: Potassium and Glucose.	Hormones that Increase Blood Glucose "STENGG" • Somatotropin (growth hormone) • Thyroid hormones (thyroxine and triiodothyronine) • Epinephrine • Norepinephrine
TIRED • Tachycardia • Irritability • Restlessness • Excessive Hunger • Diaphoresis Rhyme Cold and clammy, need some	3 P's • Polyphagia • Polydipsia • Polyuria Rhyme Hot and dry, sugar high

Hisutism—The 5 Hs 5 Hs	Attenuated (live/weakened) Vaccines "ROME Is My Best Place To Yell!"
Multiple Myeloma Symptoms CRAB:	White Blood Cells (In order of decreasing numbers.) "Nobody Likes My Educational Background" or "Never Let Monkeys Eat Bananas"

<table>
<tr>
<td>

"ROME Is My Best Place To Yell!"
- Rubella
- Oral polio vaccine
- Measles
- Epidemic typhus
- Influenza
- Mumps
- BCG

</td>
<td>

5 Hs
- Hirsutism
- Hyperplasia of gums
- Harm to kidneys
- Hypertension
- Hyperglycemia

</td>
</tr>
<tr>
<td>

- Neutrophils
- Lymphocytes
- Monocytes
- Eosinophils
- Basophils

</td>
<td>

CRAB:
- Calcium level elevated
- Renal failure
- Anemia
- Bone breakdown and resorption

</td>
</tr>
</table>

<table>
<tr>
<td>

AIDS—The Cells Attacked

</td>
<td>

Cancer's Early Warning Signs
CAUTION UP

</td>
</tr>
<tr>
<td>

Melanoma Characteristics
ABCDE

</td>
<td>

Burns—Rule of Nines and
Rule of Palms
Total body surface area
(TBSA): Rule of Nines:

</td>
</tr>
</table>

•Change bowel/bladder •A lesion doesnt heal •Unusual bleeding/discharge •Thickening/lump breast/elsewhere •Indigestion/difficulty swallowing •Obvious change wart/mole •Nagging cough/persistent	AIDS—The Cells Attacked AIDS is 4 letters long. AIDS attacks CD4 T cells.
• 9% Head • 9% Chest • 9% Abdomen • 9% Upper back • 9% Lower back	ABCDE • Asymmetrical • Borders irregular • Color dark and variation • Diameter is large (> 6MM) • Evolving

<table>
<tr><td>

Scleroderma
CREST syndrome:

</td><td>

Syphilis—Primary
PRESS

</td></tr>
<tr><td>

Syphilis—Tertiary
CLASS

</td><td>

Syphilis—Secondary
CAMP

</td></tr>
</table>

PRESS	CREST syndrome:
• Painless lesion • Regional lymphadenopathy • Exudate • Single lesion • Sexual contact can cause	• Calcinosis • Raynaud's Syndrome • Esophageal Motility Disorder • Sclerodactyly • Telangiectasia
CAMP • Condyloma lata • Acute Infection symptoms (fever, sore throat, malaise, weight loss) • Mucocutaneous lesion, mucous patches • Papules & Pustules	**CLASS** • Cardiovascular disorder • Late benign syphilis (gumma) • Asymptomatic Neurosyphilis • Symptomatic Neurosyphilis

<table>
<tr>
<td>

Sprains and
Strains—Interventions
RICE

</td>
<td>

Traction Care
TRACTION

</td>
</tr>
<tr>
<td>

Autonomic Nervous System
Functions Rhyme

</td>
<td>

Canes and Walkers
COAL and WWAL

</td>
</tr>
</table>

TRACTION • Temperature (Extremity, Infection) • hang freely • Alignment • Circulation Check (5 P's) • Type & Location of fracture • Increase fluide intake • Overhead trapeze	RICE • Rest • Ice • Compression • Elevation
COAL • Cane • Opposite • Affected • Leg WWAL • Walker • With	Sympathetic: fight or flight Parasympathetic: rest and digest

Prioritization The order in which we use the strategies in a priority question: PHAN	Nursing Process How to find the correct answer by using the nursing process. Assess before you implement! ADPIE:
Inflammation—Signs PRISH	Patient Handoff Report I-SBAR patient handoff reporting supports the National Patient Safety Goal #2, "to improve effectiveness of communication among caregivers."

Assess before you implement! ADPIE: •Assessment •Diagnosis •Planning •Implementation •Evaluation	PHAN •Priority •Hierarchy •ABCs •Nursing Process
I-SBAR: •Identify •Situation •Background •Assessment •Recommendation	PRISH • Pain • Redness • Immobility (loss of function) • Swelling • Heat

Activities of Daily Living (ADL) BATTED	Instrumental Activities of Daily Living (IADL) SCUM
Gestation—Bartholomew's Rule of Fours	Oxygen Dissociation—Right Shift A right shift is a DATE with CO_2

SCUM •Shopping •Cooking and Cleaning •Using telephone or transportation •Managing money and medications	BATTED •Bathing •Ambulation •Toileting •Transfers •Eating •Dressing
A right shift is a DATE with CO_2 •2,3 Diphosphoglycerate DPG •Acidosis •Temperature •Exercise	Gestation—Bartholomew's Rule of Fours • 12 Weeks: Symphisis pubis • 16 weeks: Midway between symphysis pubis and umbilicus • 20 weeks: Umbilicus • 36 weeks: Xiphoid process

<table>
<tr><td>

Teratogens
TAP CAP

</td><td>

Clubfoot—Deformities
InAdEquate

</td></tr>
<tr><td>

Nephritic Syndrome
PHARAOH

</td><td>

Esophageal Atresia and
Tracheoesophageal Fistula
3 C's

</td></tr>
</table>

InAdEquate • Inversion • Adduction • Equinus	TAP CAP • Thalidomide • Alcohol • Progestins • Corticosteroids • Aspirin • Phenytoin
3 C's • Coughing • Choking • Cyanosis	PHARAOH • Proteinuria & Edema • Hematuria • Azotemia • RBC casts • Anti-strep titres (If post-strep) • Oliguria • Hypertension

Kidney Layers "Our Careers In Medicine"	Flow of fluid through the Kidney "Be Prepared To Look Happy During Computer-based Testing"
Nephrotic Syndrome People Have Endless Appetites	Liver Functions PUSH DoG

Flow of fluid "Be Prepared To Look Happy During Computer-based Testing" •Bowmans capsule •Proximal Tubules •Loop Henle •Distal and Convoluted Tubules	Kidney layers "Our Careers In Medicine" • Outer cortex • Inner medulla
PUSH DoG • Protein synthesis • Ureas synthesis • Storage • Hormone synthesis • Detoxification • Glucose and fat metabolism	People Have Endless Appetites • Proteinuria • Hyperlipidemia • Edema • Albuminuria & hypoalbuminemia

<table>
<tr>
<td>

Intestinal Components
Bowel Components (in order):
Dow Jones Industrial Can't
Choose Stocks

</td>
<td>

Streptococcus
pyogenes—Diseases
GET NIPPLES

</td>
</tr>
<tr>
<td>

Rubella, Congenital—Signs
"Rubber Ducky, I so Blue"

</td>
<td>

Common Cold—Causes
CREAR:

</td>
</tr>
</table>

GET NIPPLES • Glomerulonephritis • Endocarditis (Heart Valves) • Toxic shock syndrome • Necrotizing fasciitis and myositis • Impetigo • Pharyngitis • Pneumonia	Dow Jones Industrial Can't Choose Stocks • Duodenum • Jejunum • Ileum • Cecum • Colon • Sigmoid
CREAR: • Coronavirus • Rhinoviruses • Enterovirus • Adenovirus • Respiratory Syncytial Virus (RSV)	"Rubber Ducky, I so Blue" • Rubella • Patent ductus arteriosus • Eyes • Blueberry muffin rash

<table>
<tr>
<td>

Staph aureus
caused by SOFT PAINS

</td>
<td>

E. coli causes DUNG

</td>
</tr>
<tr>
<td>

Triage color system
Red, Yellow, Green, Black
32 can do

</td>
<td>

Pseudomonas Aeruginosa
P-S-E-U   &   A-E-R-U-G-I-
N-O-S-A

</td>
</tr>
</table>

E. coli causes DUNG • Diarrhea • UTI • Neonatal meningitis • Gram negative sepsis	Staph aureus caused by SOFT PAINS • Skin infections • Osteomyelitis • Food poisoning • Toxic shock syndrome • Pneumonia • Acute endocarditis • Infective arthritis
P-S-E-U •Pneumonia •Sepsis •External otits media •UTI A-E-R-U-G-I-N-O-S-A •Aerobic •Exotoxin A •Rod	Red–Don't with within 15 mins they will die, ABC problem, above 30, no pulse, mentally confused Yellow–30 mins, not ABC but still wounded, above 30, pulse, mental status normal Green–emotional issues, walking wounded

heat vs cold first	Walking Up and Down stairs with crutches
Stages of Labor	Naegele's rule

Good people go to heaven (good leg up) Bad people go to hell (bad leg down)	Use heat first for muscles Use cold first for nerves
1st day of LMP - 3 months (don't forget to adjust year if needed) + 7 days (don't forget to adjust the month if needed)	1. Getting ready to Push a. Latent – 0-3, little to no pain b. Active – 3-7, c. Transition – 7-10, effacement 100% 2. Pushing = Baby 3. Placenta 4. Bonding

Postpartum Lochia changes	Decels and Accels (FHR) Change> Cause> What to do VEAL >CHOP> MINE
Parkland Formula (Fluid Replacement) for Burns	PROM vs. PPROM

Variable Dec>Cord compression>Move(Trendelen burg>Csection) Early Dec>Head Compression>Identify Labor(active good, no progression bad) Accel>OK>Nothing Late Dec>Placenta	Rubra (3-5 days, blood & clots) Serosa (10 days, pink) Alba (up to 2-5 weeks, Should not be longer than 6 weeks, white/creamy)
*PROM(Premature Rupture of Membrane) = More than 1 hour before onset of labor, Use Pitocin to get things moving *PPROM (Preterm)= 37 weeks and More than 1 hour before onset of labor, Risk for infection (prophylactic ATB), Bed Rest, Steroids (if needed)	[4 x wgt (kg) x TBSA %] / 2 = ANSWER ANSWER – give in first 8 hours ANSWER – give in next 16 hours

Mnemonics
Crosswords

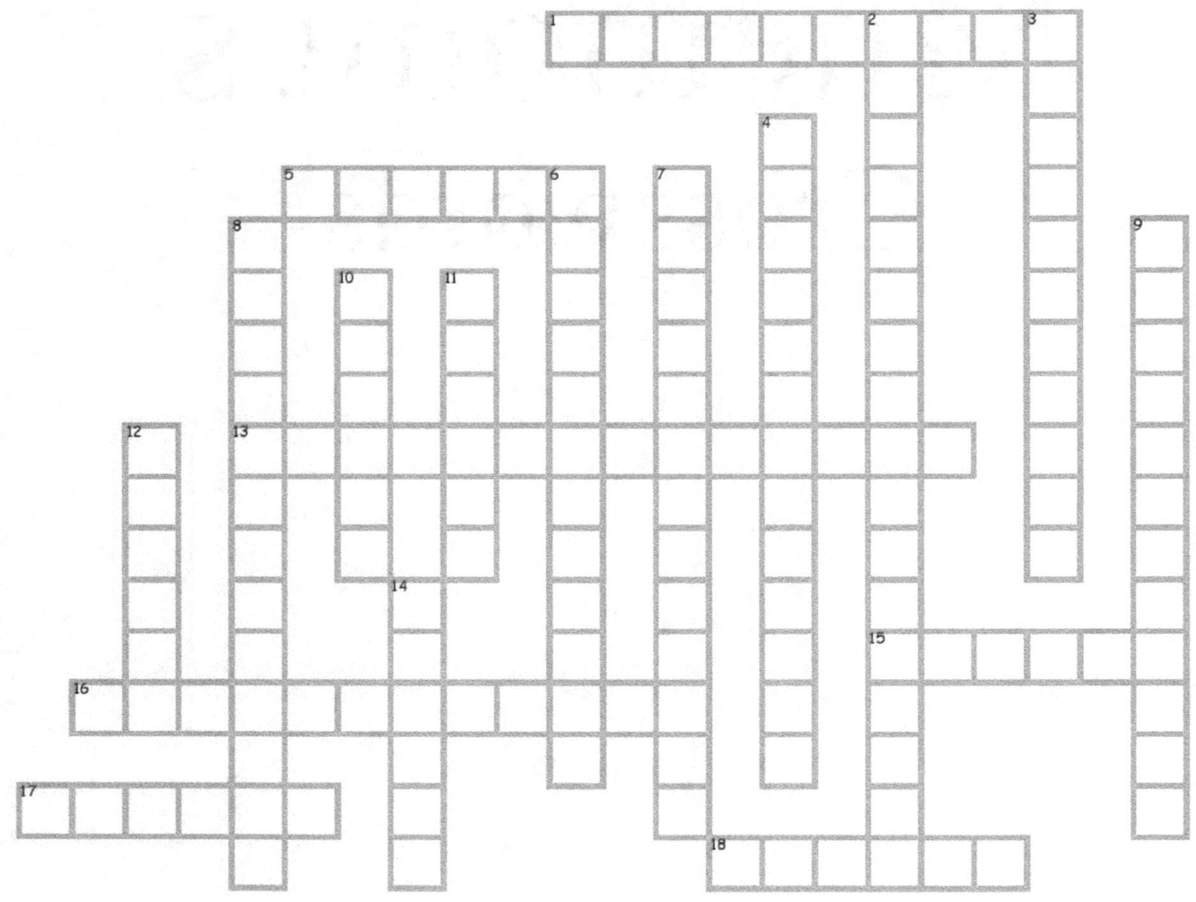

Across

1. K- Kayexalate (orally/ enema) I- Insulin N- Na HCO3 D- Diuretics (____ & Thiazides)
5. T-achycardia I-rritability R-estless E-xcessive ____ D-iaphoresis/ Depression
13. A-ssessment A-nanlysis P-lanning ____ E-valuation
15. Anticholingergics Side Effects: 4-____
16. B- Brain Damage A- Alcoholic ____ D- Death
17. S-leep Disturbances I-nterest Decreased ____ Feelings
18. A-irway ____ I-ncreased Pulse R-estlessness R-etractions A-nxiety Increased I-nspiratory Stridor D-rooling

Down

2. S-ugar (Glucocorticoids) S-alt (____) S-ex (Androgens)
3. Promotion of Normal ____ (POOPER SCOOP)
4. I - ____ D - Dopamine E - Epinephrine A - Atropine Sulfate
6. Early Hypoxia: ____ A-nxiety T-achycardia/ Tachypnea Late Hypoxia: B-radycardia E-xtreme Restlessness D-yspnea
7. C - Convulsions A- ____ - Tetany S - Spasms and stridor
8. Tremor Heart rate up Yawning (fatigueability) Restlessness Oligomenorrhea & amenorrhea Intolerance to heat Diarrhea ____ Sweating Muscle wasting & weight loss
9. 4 C's of ____ (Complications)
10. C-hoking L-ie on back E-valuate Airway F-eed Slowly T-eaching L-arger ____ opening I-ncidence incerase in males P-revent crust formation and aspiration
11. Osteoporosis Risk Factors (____)
12. B-reasts U-terus B-owels B-ladder ____ E-pisiotomy/lateration/C-section incision
14. Complications of Trauma ____ (TRAUMATIC)

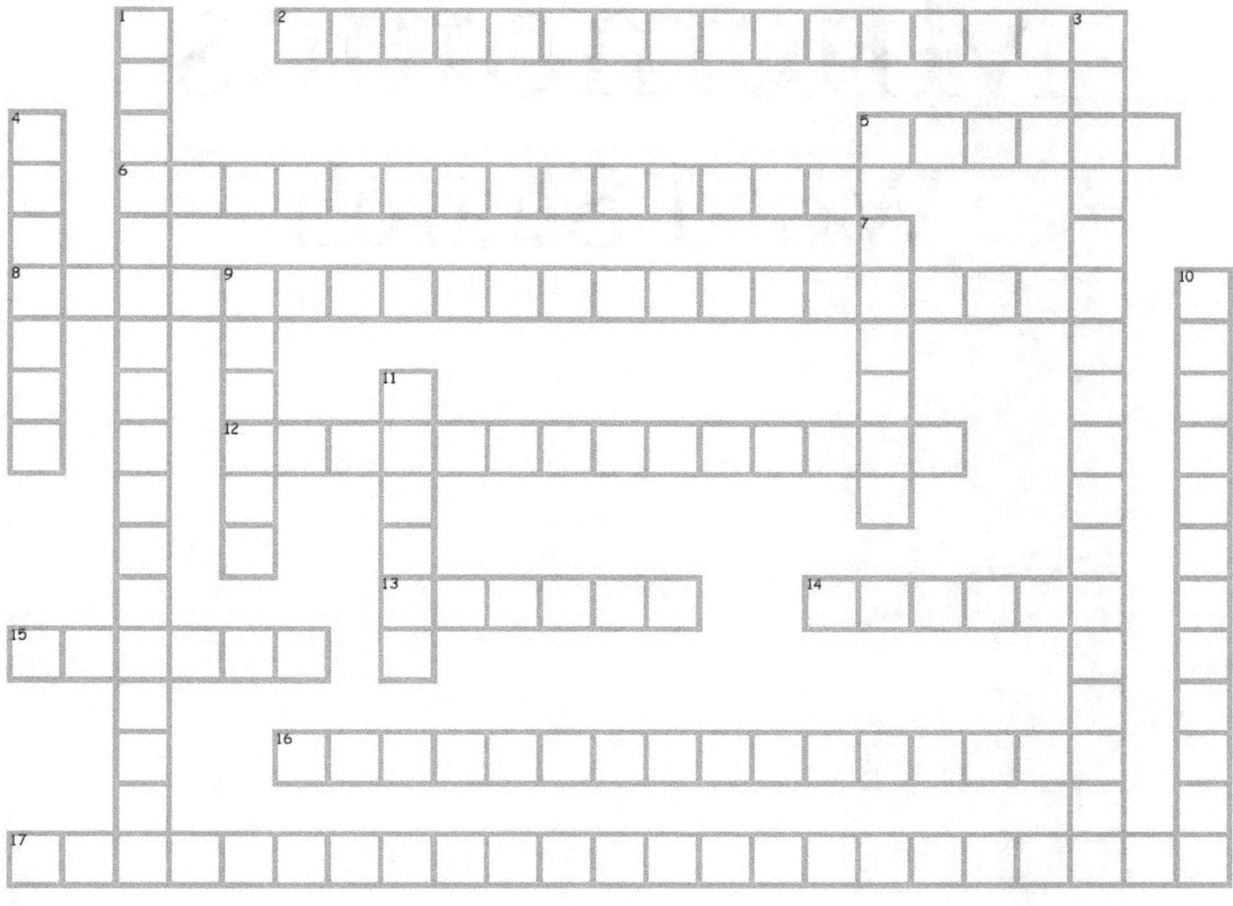

Across

2 INsulIN stimulates 2 things to go IN 2 _____ and Glucose.
5 Activities of Daily _____ (ADL) BATTED
6 Nursing Process How to find the correct answer by using the nursing _____ before you implement! ADPIE:
8 Melanoma _____
12 TIRED • Tachycardia • _____ Restlessness • Excessive Hunger • Diaphoresis Rhyme Cold and clammy, need some candy
13 Rubra (3-5 days, blood & clots) Serosa (10 days, pink) Alba (up to 2-5 weeks, _____ not be longer than 6 weeks, white/creamy)
14 Cranial nerves order "Oh, oh, oh, to touch and feel a girl's _____. Such heaven!"
15 Cranial nerves : S: sensory; m: motor; b: both "Some say marry money but my brother says big brains _____ more"
16 Nephritic _____
17 6 Ps _____ Bronchial Constriction •Possible Foreign Body •Pulmonary Embolus •Pneumothorax •Pump Failure

Down

1 PRESS • Painless lesion • Regional _____ Exudate • Single lesion • Sexual contact can cause
3 Asthma _____:
4 CRAB: • _____ level elevated • Renal failure • Anemia • Bone breakdown and resorption
7 CAMP • Condyloma _____ Acute Infection symptoms (fever, sore throat, malaise, weight loss) • Mucocutaneous lesion, mucous patches • Papules & Pustules
9 1. Getting ready to Push a. Latent – 0-3, little to no pain b. _____ – 3-7, c. Transition – 7-10, effacement 100% 2. Pushing = Baby 3. Placenta 4. Bonding
10 "CPR" • _____ Stage • Progressive Stage • Refractory Stage
11 Sympathetic: fight or flight Parasympathetic: rest and _____

Mnemonics
Word Search

Nursing Mnemonics Word Search Puzzle

```
G U A R D S D S D M P P U L S E Z B N U T R I T I O N H F L S F P W P
S Q E J Z A V E C G A D J W E U A Z M O S S N V R G Y L L G Z L Q R A
S T Z Y M W M A N R E N A S T A N E P C I E I E N R P C U A N M P H R
E Q P A I E I I E S T D T A X I S P S J Q P I S E R D Z I X M A F E T
N T G A N D T D A X N E K L M T I T M Y L F Z R Y M L P D T B I Q U I
D E J J A R A E T I E K L M T I C E N T R A L F M L L D S U I F X M A
N U I A E U R R N I I I L U T E G P B J T I V Z P D A E V E N T S A L
I A C W O C K E E K L U U T T E G C Z Z P A C C E S S I S L S Y W T M
L F S H N T E G N M W C S E G F I H R I U E T G F J S E D W U K E I A
B ▢ S I N T S N S F L I G H T B L Y D A N E M I A E Y K O O L C I C I
F E V E R ▢ T U S E A N O M : T N E M E G A N A M I M J V R I N G A M
O D D V J T U H E L E V A T E D M Y A N A G N I R E D N A W N F H B I
S D Y M O T O I S I P E D E R I T : A I M E C Y L G O P Y H S O T F L
P I D E P R E S S I O N O Y A T A T B R O T H E R L L Y L I W L M K U
3 D I S T U R B A N C E S L I C I R C U L A T I O N E N I M A P O D B
```

- ☐ CARDIAC
- ☐ ASSESSMENT
- ☐ N-UTRITION
- ☐ E-VENTS
- ☐ ACCESS
- ☐ CLIENT
- ☐ CIRCULATION
- ☐ NEEDLES
- ☐ MONROE
- ☐ RHEUMATIC
- ☐ HUNGER
- ☐ BULIMIA
- ☐ EPISIOTOMY
- ☐ GUARDS
- ☐ DEMENTIA
- ☐ MELLITUS
- ☐ INCREASED
- ☐ WANDERING
- ☐ BROTHER
- ☐ O-PPOSITE
- ☐ HYPERLIPIDEMIA
- ☐ DIALYSIS
- ☐ HYPOGLYCEMIA: TIRED
- ☐ FLIGHT
- ☐ CENTRAL
- ☐ M-ANAGING
- ☐ A-NXIETY
- ☐ ANEMIA
- ☐ LEVATED
- ☐ LITTLE
- ☐ INSULIN
- ☐ P-PULSE
- ☐ DAMAGE
- ☐ FEVER▢T
- ☐ DEPRESSION
- ☐ MAXIMAL
- ☐ DISTURBANCES
- ☐ ▢SWEATING
- ☐ 3 P'S OF BLINDNESS
- ☐ SHOULDER
- ☐ MI MANAGEMENT: MONA
- ☐ PARTIAL
- ☐ WEIGHT
- ☐ INCREASED
- ☐ FLUIDS
- ☐ DOPAMINE

Mnemonics for NCLEX Word Search Puzzle

```
T E R A T O G E N S   T A P C A P L Q W M M E M L Q C A J A F R S U V
• R Y M P O M X X • W Q Y Z C N J I G X Y B A A N • B • E T • A
  M A D I O H O C E S S E P G J S W O F O T N H E D   • M T U N U G E R
E • V L P R O C N J S N K S N U S Q P   R G R N Y O A I E I S S E R I
N M F U A T C I O J B T S H A A V U I E A S E O R N E D   D N T E O T A
I K E S I P S A S O H A M K N E • P Y L L O T H I R S T I U Y U C F G A B
R T Z A I O J B T R E L R P M E • P Y A D G T P O N O E D   • S S C L F A R I
H I R F Z A L T R E A W M E • E G   E E L A R E
P S P Z C A B E R A M T L R E • E G • E E L A R E
E R V D K Z T O N A M T P T E L V I O S H A P O L Y D I P S I A D H R N I A O H G L
N E Q L X U I E L T P T E T I O S H A P C " S E G A T S — K C O H E R N N E B P M E
I V A V P D R K V I J E T I L L H " R P C " S E G A T S O N E D A H P M Y L T
P N V M S D C V U U S L L H " R P C   Y H T A P O N E D A H P M Y L G L R
D C A L U M R O F N O I T U A C   S N G I S D I S O R D E R   • H P R
```

□ SHOULD	□ ALKALOSIS •	□ SHOCK—STAGES "CPR"
□ NAEGELE'S RULE	□ SEPSIS	□ PARTICULAR
□ ABDUCENS CN	□ JANEWAY	□ CAREERS
□ STEROIDS	□ LYMPHADENOPATHY •	□ COMPUTER-BASED
□ LETTERS	□ A •ROD •UTI	□ TELEPHONE
□ STAGES OF LABOR	□ PROGRESSION	□ STOCKS •
□ SIGNS CAUTION	□ TEMPERATURE •	□ VARIATION •
□ WITHIN	□ DISORDER •	□ ANEMIA •
□ INFECTION) •	□ TERATOGENS TAP CAP	□ POLYDIPSIA
□ METABOLISM	□ SYMPTOMS	□ EPINEPHRINE •
□ FORMULA	□ DIGEST	□ DRUGS/DIET •
□ XIPHOID	□ THIRST	□ KIDNEYS •
□ INVERSION •	□ WALKER •	□ PROCESS
□ IV) •MASK	□ ADRENAL	

Mnemonics
Matching

Nursing Mnemonics Matching

Write the code corresponding to the correct match in the space provided.

____ 1. To apply a telemetry monitor:

____ 2. HYPOGLYCEMIA: TIRED

____ 3. 5W's of common causes of post-op fever

____ 4. Assess Changes in Senile Dementia (JAMCO)

____ 5. Hyperkalemia Management (KIND)

____ 6. Assessment Tests for Fetal Well-Being (ALONE)

____ 7. Energy Decreased (CAPS)

____ 8. Post-Partum Assessment (BUBBLE)

____ 9. OB Non-Stress Test (NNN) 3 negatives in a row to interpret results of Non-Stress Test

____ 10. Management of Myocardial Infarction (MONATAS)

____ 11. Acid-Base (ROME)

____ 12. Symptoms of Hypoxia (RAT BED)

____ 13. Trauma Surgery (AMPLE) after initial assessment

____ 14. 5 D's of Behavioral Problems of Alcoholism

____ 15. Outcome of Alcoholism: BAD

____ 16. Canes and Walkers (COAL)

____ 17. Major Symptoms of a Manic Attack (DIG

A1. T- Tetralogy of Fallot T- Truncus Arteriosus T- Transportation of the Great Vessels T- Tricuspid Atresia

B1. D-elirium I-nfection A-trophic Urethra P-harmaceuticals P-sychologic E-xcess Urine Output R-estricted Mobility S-tool Impaction

C1. B-athing A-mbulation T-oileting T-ransfers E-ating D-ressing

D1. A-irway B-reathing C-irculation D-isability E-xamine F-ahrenheit G-et Vitals H-ead to Toe Assessment I-ntervention

E1. S-ugar (Glucocorticoids) S-alt (Mineralcorticoids) S-ex (Androgens)

F1. R- Razor Electric/ Blades A- Aspirin N- No needles (esp. in small gauge) D- Do decrease in needle sticks) I - Injury (Protect from)

G1. M - Muscle weakness U - Urine, oliguria, anuria R- Respiratory distress D - Decreased cardiac contractility E - ECG changes R - Reflexes, hyperreflexia, or areflexia (flaccid)

H1. F - Frequency (3x per week) I - Intensity (60-80% of Maximal Heart Rate) T- Time (Aerobic Activity)

I1. T-achycardia I-rritability R-estless E-xcessive Hunger D-iaphoresis/ Depression

J1. A- Acid-Base Problems E- Electrolyte Problems I- Intoxications O- Overload of fluids U - Uremic Symptoms

K1. P-Pain P-Paresthesia P-Paralysis P-Pulse P-Pallor (Paleness)

L1. K- Kayexalate (orally/ enema) I- Insulin N- Na HCO3 D- Diuretics (Furosemide & Thiazides)

M1. A-drenergics (Albuterol) S-teroids T-heophylline H-ydration (IV) M-ask (Oxygen) A-ntibiotics

N1. P- Preventable P- Painless P- Permanent

O1. A-ssessment D- iagnosis P-lanning I-mplementation E-valuaton

P1. A- Amniocentesis L- L/S Ratio O - Oxytocin Test N - Non-Stress Test E - Estriol Level

Q1. B- Banana R- Rice A- Apple T- Toasted Bread

R1. S-lurred Speech A-ltered Central Nervous System M-uscle Twitching S-eizures

S1. A-llergies M-edications P-ast Medical History L-ast Meal E-vents Surrounding Injury

T1. Can't see Can't pee Can't spit Can't sh*t

U1. A- Anemia N- Neutropenia T- Thrombocytopenia

V1. P-osition O-utput O-ffer Fluids P-rivacy E-xercise R-eport Results S-ize (Amount) C-onsistency O-ccult Blood O-dor P-eristalsis

W1. P- Pulmonary Bronchial Constriction P- Possible Foreign Body

FAST)

_____ 18. 3 P's of Blindness

_____ 19. Eating Disorder: ANOREXIA

_____ 20. Hypoglycemia (TIRED) - an abnormal decrease of blood in the sugar

_____ 21. Steps in the Nursing Process ADPIE (A Delicious PIE)

_____ 22. Cranial Nerve Mnemonic 01

_____ 23. Epiglottitis (AIR RAID)

_____ 24. PUPIL SIZE miotic & mydriatic

_____ 25. DEMENTIA

_____ 26. Prostate Problems are no... FUN

_____ 27. Osteoporosis Risk Factors (ACCESS)

_____ 28. TDCI (These Drugs Can Interact)

_____ 29. Canes and Walkers (WWAL) Wandering Wilma's Always Late

_____ 30. Evalution of Episiotomy Healing (REEDA)

_____ 31. HYPERNATREMIA "You Are Fried"

_____ 32. 6 P's of Dyspnea

_____ 33. Tracheal Esophageal Fistula (3 C's)

_____ 34. Anticholingergics Side Effects: 4-CAN'Ts

_____ 35. CANCER Interventions

_____ 36. Who needs dialysis? (Check the vowels: AEIOU)

_____ 37. Emergency Trauma Assessment (ABCDEFGHI)

_____ 38. Cranial Nerve

P- Pulmonary Embolus P- Pneumothorax P- Pump Failure P- Pneumonia

X1. T-issue Perfusion Problems R-espiratory Problems A-nxiety U-nstable Clotting Factors M-alnutrition A-ltered Body Image T-hromboembolism I-nfection C-oping Problems

Y1. C- Coronary Artery Disease C- Coronary Rheumatic Fever C- Congestive Heart Failure C- Cardio Vascular Accident

Z1. Change in bowel/bladder A lesion doesn't heal Unusual bleeding/discharge Thickening lump in breast/elsewhere Indigestion/difficulty swallowing Obvious changes wart/mole Nagging cough/persistent hoarseness Unexplained weight loss Pernicious Anemia

A2. S- Some S- Say M - Marry M- Money B- But M- My B - Brother S- Says B- Bad B- Business M - Marry M - Money

B2. D- Denial D- Dependency D- Demanding D- Destructive D- Domineering

C2. O- On O -Old O- Obando T- Tower T- Top A- F- Filipino A - Army G - Guards V - Villages A - And H - Huts

D2. Amenorrhea delayed No organic factors accounts for weight loss Obviously thin but feels FAT Refusal to maintain normal body weight Epigastric discomfort is common Xsymptoms (peculiar symptoms) Intense fears of gaining weight Always thinking of foods

E2. W-eight loss of 15% of original body weight A-menorrhea S-ocial withdrawal H-istory of high activity & achievement E-lectrolyte Imbalance D-epression/ Distorted Body Image

F2. P- Potassium I- Inside S- Sodium O- Outside

G2. C- Cough H- Hemoptysis O- Orthopnea P- Pulmonary Congestion (crackles/ rales)

H2. H- emolysis E- levated L- iver function tests L- ow P- latelet count

I2. Make sure they don't have problems with: D-rug and alcohol E-yes and ears M-etabolic and endocrine disorders E-motional disorders N-eurologic disorders T-umors and trauma I-nfection A-rteriovascular disease

J2. T - Theophyline D - Dilantin C - Coumadin I - Iosone (Erythromycin)

K2. R- Rye O- Oats W- Wheat

L2. S Stenosis P Partial obstruction A Aneurysms S Septal defect M Mitral regurgitation

M2. H-eat I-nduration P-ain E-dema R-edness

N2. C-oncentration decreased A-ppetite P-sychomotor function decreased S-uicidal Ideations

O2. M-Morphine A-Aminophylline D- Digitalis D-Diuretics (Lasix) O- Oxygen G- ases (Blood Gases ABG's)

P2. White over right (top right shoulder) Black beside the white (Over lt shoulder) Checkers (red below the black) Christmas

Mnemonic 03

___ 39. Complications of Trauma Client (TRAUMATIC)

___ 40. Inflammation (HIPER)

___ 41. Bleeding Precautions (RANDI)

___ 42. Hyperthyroidism (s/s) : THYROIDISM

___ 43. Promotion of Normal Elimination (POOPER SCOOP)

___ 44. MI management: MONA

___ 45. Cranial Nerve Mnemonic 02

___ 46. 3 P's of Diabetes Mellitus - Type 1 Signs & Symptoms

___ 47. Steps in the Nursing Process AAPIE (An Apple Pie)

___ 48. HEART MURMURS: SPASM

___ 49. Cranial Nerve Mnemonics 02 (Sensory, Motor or Both)

___ 50. Left-Sided Heart Failure (CHOP)

___ 51. Treating CHF (UNLOAD FAST)

___ 52. Nursing Care for Sprains and Strains (RICE)

___ 53. Depression Assessment (SIG)

___ 54. Findings of a Bulimia client: WASHED

___ 55. Hypertension Nursing Care (DIURETIC)

___ 56. Severe Pre-Eclampsia (HELLP)

___ 57. Cleft Lip - Post Op Care (CLEFT LIP)

(Green beside the red) Then ofcourse, the brown will be in the middle!

Q2. B- Brain Damage A- Alcoholic Hallucinosis D- Death

R2. C-hoking L-ie on back E-valuate Airway F-eed Slowly T-eaching L-arger nipple opening I-ncidence increase in males P-revent crust formation and aspiration

S2. A- Abdominal Pain C - Chest Pain H - Headache E - Eye Problems S - Severe Leg Pain

T2. A-mnesia A-nomia A-praxia A-gnosia A-phasia

U2. SALT S = Skin flushed A = Agitation L = Low-grade fever T = Thirst

V2. Tremor Heart rate up Yawning (fatigueability) Restlessness Oligomenorrhea & amenorrhea Intolerance to heat Diarrhea Irritability Sweating Muscle wasting & weight loss

W2. R- Redness E- Edema E - Ecchymosis D - Discharge, Drainage A - Approximation

X2. S-hopping C-ooking and Cleaning U-sing telephone or transportaiton M-anaging money and medications

Y2. S - Some S - Says M- Marilyn M- Monroe B - But M- My B- Brother S- Says B- Bridget B - Bardot M- Mmm M- Mmm

Z2. T-ricuspid P-ulmonic M-itrial A-ortic

A3. U-pright Position N-itrates (in low dose) L-asix O-xygen A-minophylline D-igoxin F-luids (decrease) A-fterload (decrease) S-odium restriction T-est (Dig level, ABGs, K level)

B3. Early Hypoxia: R-estlessness A-nxiety T-achycardia/ Tachypnea Late Hypoxia: B-radycardia E-xtreme Restlessness D-yspnea

C3. W- Walker W- With A- Affected L - Leg

D3. C- Cane O- Opposite A- Affected L- Leg

E3. T Tired I Irritability R Restless E Excessive hunger D Diaphoresis-Depression

F3. A-llergies M-edications P-ast Medical History L-ast Meal E-vents Surrounding Injury

G3. R-espiratory O-pposite M-etabolic E-qual

H3. P- Polyuria (excessive urination) P- Polydypsia (excessive thirst) P- Polyphagia (excessive hunger)

I3. S-lurred Speech A-ltered Central Nervous System M-uscle Twitching S-eizures

J3. M - Medications - ACE inhibitors, NSAIDS A - Acidosis - Metabolic and respiratory C - Cellular destruction - Burns, traumatic injury H - Hypoaldosteronism, hemolysis I - Intake - Excesssive N - Nephrons, renal failure E - Excretion - Impaired

K3. B-inge eating U-nder strict dieting L-acks control over-eating I-nduced vomiting M-inimum of to binge eating episodes I-ncrease/Persistent concern of body size/shape A-buse of diuretics & laxatives

___ 58. CANCER'S Early Warning Signs CAUTION UP

___ 59. Exercise Guide for Diabetic Fitness (FIT)

___ 60. Cyanotic Defects: 4 T's

___ 61. Electrolytes - PISO

___ 62. "CATS" of "HYPOCALCEMIA"

___ 63. Symptoms of Hypoxia (in Pediatrics) - FINES

___ 64. Pulmonary Edema (MAD DOG)

___ 65. Signs and Symptoms of Increased Serum K+: MURDER

___ 66. BRAT Diet (for severe dehydration)

___ 67. 5 A's to Alzheimer Diagnosis

___ 68. Care of Client in Traction (TRACTION)

___ 69. 5 P's of Circulatory Checks

___ 70. Common Causes of Transient Incontinence (DIAPPERS)

___ 71. Emergency Drugs to LEAN on

___ 72. The HYPERKALEMIA "Machine" - Causes of Increased Serum K+

___ 73. IADLS (Instrumental Activities of Daily Living) SCUM

___ 74. Right-Sided Heart Failure (HEAD)

___ 75. Acute Pancreatitis: I GET SMASHED

___ 76. Trauma Surgery (AMPLE) after initial

L3. S-leep Disturbances I-nterest Decreased G-uilty Feelings

M3. L- Lidocaine E - Epinephrine A- Atropine Sulfate N - Narcan

N3. A-lcohol Use C-orticosteroid Use C-alcium low E-strogen low S-moking S-edentary lifestyle/s ACCESS leads to OSTEOPOROSIS

O3. D-aily Weight I- ntake and Output (I & O) U- rine Output R-esponse of BP E-lectrolytes T-ake Pulses I-schemic Episodes (TIA) C-omplications: 4C's

P3. O- Oh O- Oh O- Oh T- To T- Touch A- And F - Feel A G - irl's V - agina S - So H- Heavenly

Q3. F-eeding difficulty I-nspiratory Stridor N-ares Flares E-xpiratory Grunting S-ternal Retractions

R3. N - Non-reactive N - Non- Stress is N - Not good

S3. I - Isoproterenol D - Dopamine E - Epinephrine A - Atropine Sulfate

T3. R- Ruthless A- Abusive P- Personal E- Experience

U3. Child's excessive knowledge on sex & abusive words Hair growth in various lengths Inconsistent stories from the child & parent/s Low self-esteem Depression Apathy, no emotion Bruised Unusual injuries Serious injuries Evidence of old injuries not reported

V3. Idiopathic Gallstone E - EtOH Trauma Steroids Mumps (paramyxovirus) and other viruses (EBV, CMV) Autoimmune Scorpion sting / snake bite H ypercalcemia, hyperlipidemia and hypothermia E - ERCP Drugs, duodenal ulcers

W3. C- Choking C- Coughing C - Cyanosis

X3. A-irway Closed I-ncreased Pulse R-estlessness R-etractions A-nxiety Increased I-nspiratory Stridor D-rooling

Y3. Miotic: Little word=Little pupil Mydriatic: Big word=Big pupil

Z3. C-omfort A-ltered Body Image N-utrition C-hemotherapy E-valuate response to meds R-espite for caretakers

A4. Morphine O2 Nitroglycerine Aspirin

B4. OLympic (Olfactory) OPium (Optic) OCcupies (Oculomotor) TROubled (Trochlear) TRIathletes (Trigeminal) After (Abducens) Finishing (Facial) VEgas (Vestibulocochlear) Gambling (Glossopharyngeal) VAcations (Vagus) Still (Spinal Accessory) High (Hypoglossal)

C4. J- Judgment A- Affect M- Memory C- Cognition O- Orientation

D4. F- Frequency U- Urgency N- Nocturia

E4. D- Distractibility I - Indiscretion G - Grandiosity F- Flight of Ideas A- Activity Increase S- Sleep Deficit T - Talkative

F4. B-reasts U-terus B-owels B-ladder L-ochia E-pisiotomy/lateration/C-section incision

G4. M- Morphine O- Oxygen N- Nitrates (Nitroglycerin) A- Aspirin (ASA) T- Thormbolytics A- Anti-Coagulants S- Stool Softeners

H4. R- Rest I - Ice C - Compression E- Elevation

assessment

___ 77. Situations requiring Crisis Situation: RAPE

___ 78. Eating Disorder: BULIMIA

___ 79. Warning Signs of a Child Abuse/ Neglect: CHILD ABUSE

___ 80. Lidocaine Toxicity (SAMS)

___ 81. Management of ASTHMA

___ 82. 4 C's of Hypertension (Complications)

___ 83. Drugs for Bradycardia & low BP (IDEA)

___ 84. Adrenal Gland Hormones (SSS)

___ 85. Gluten Free Diet (ROW)

___ 86. Serious Complications of Oral Birth Control Pills (ACHES)

___ 87. Cholinergic Crisis (SLUD)

___ 88. Blood Flow Through the Cardiac Valves (Tissue Paper My Assets)

___ 89. Evalution of Episiotomy Healing (REEDA)

___ 90. ADLs (Activity of Daily Living) BATTED

___ 91. Lidocaine Toxicity (SAMS)

___ 92. Immediate Treatment of a Myocardial Infarction Client (MONA)

___ 93. Cranial Nerve Mnemonics (Sensory, Motor or Both)

I4. Wind (think pneumonia, splinting, incentive spirometer exercises not done, DB+ coughing not done) Water (dehydration...) Wound (infection, dehiscence...) Walking (PE...) Wonder drug (approriate antibiotic...)

J4. R- Redness E- Edema E - Ecchymosis D - Discharge, Drainage A - Approximation

K4. A-ssessment A-nanlysis P-lanning I-mplementation E-valuation

L4. S-alivation L-acrimation U-rination D-efecation

M4. M- Morphine O- Oxygen N- Nitroglycerine A- ASA

N4. C - Convulsions A- Arrhythmias T - Tetany S - Spasms and stridor

O4. F - Fever (low grade), flushed skin R - Restless (irritable) I - Increased fluid retention and increased BP E - Edema (peripheral and pitting) D - Decreased urinary output, dry mouth

P4. H- Hepatomegaly E- Edema (Bipedal) A- Ascites D- Distended Neck Vein

Q4. T- Temperature (Extremity, Infection) R - Ropes hang freely A - Alignment C - Circulation Check (5 P's) T- Type & Location of fracture I - Increase fluide intake O - Overhead trapeze N - No weights on bed or floor

___ 94. Symptoms of
       Leukemia (ANT)
___ 95. HYPERNATREMIA

Mnemonics for NCLEX Matching

Write the code corresponding to the correct match in the space provided.

_____ 1. Syphilis—Primary PRESS

_____ 2. Endocarditis signs FROM JANE

_____ 3. Postpartum Lochia changes

_____ 4. Rubella, Congenital—Signs "Rubber Ducky, I so Blue"

_____ 5. Multiple Myeloma Symptoms CRAB:

_____ 6. Blood Glucose—Hormonal Influence Hormones that Increase Blood Glucose "STENGG"

_____ 7. Flow of fluid through the Kidney "Be Prepared To Look Happy During Computer-based Testing"

_____ 8. Hyperglycemia 3 P's

_____ 9. Attenuated (live/weakened) Vaccines "ROME Is My Best Place To Yell!"

_____ 10. Staph aureus caused by SOFT PAINS

_____ 11. Stages of Labor

_____ 12. Autonomic Nervous System Functions Rhyme

_____ 13. Bipolar Mania Symptoms

_____ 14. Asthma Management ASTHMA:

_____ 15. E. coli causes DUNG

_____ 16. Inflammation—Signs PRISH

_____ 17. Nephrotic Syndrome People Have Endless Appetites

_____ 18. Patient Handoff Report I-SBAR patient handoff reporting supports the National Patient Safety Goal #2, "to improve effectiveness of communication among caregivers."

A1. 3 P's • Polyphagia • Polydipsia • Polyuria Rhyme Hot and dry, sugar high

B1. TRACTION • Temperature (Extremity, Infection) • hang freely • Alignment • Circulation Check (5 P's) • Type & Location of fracture • Increase fluide intake • Overhead trapeze • No weights on bed or floor

C1. "ROME Is My Best Place To Yell!" • Rubella • Oral polio vaccine • Measles • Epidemic typhus • Influenza • Mumps • BCG • Plague • Typhoid oral vaccine • Yellow fever

D1. PRESS • Painless lesion • Regional lymphadenopathy • Exudate • Single lesion • Sexual contact can cause

E1. PHAN •Priority •Hierarchy •ABCs •Nursing Process

F1. ASTHMA: •Adrenergics (Albuterol) •Steroids •Theophylline •Hydration (IV) •Mask (Oxygen) •Antibiotics (Infection)

G1. TAP CAP • Thalidomide • Alcohol • Progestins • Corticosteroids • Aspirin • Phenytoin

H1. Dow Jones Industrial Can't Choose Stocks • Duodenum • Jejunum • Ileum • Cecum • Colon • Sigmoid

I1. 1st day of LMP - 3 months (don't forget to adjust year if needed) + 7 days (don't forget to adjust the month if needed)

J1. TIRED • Tachycardia • Irritability • Restlessness • Excessive Hunger • Diaphoresis Rhyme Cold and clammy, need some candy

K1. *PROM(Premature Rupture of Membrane) = More than 1 hour before onset of labor, Use Pitocin to get things moving *PPROM (Preterm)= 37 weeks and More than 1 hour before onset of labor, Risk for infection (prophylactic ATB), Bed Rest, Steroids (if needed)

L1. 3 C's • Coughing • Choking • Cyanosis

M1. Rubra (3-5 days, blood & clots) Serosa (10 days, pink) Alba (up to 2-5 weeks, Should not be longer than 6 weeks, white/creamy)

N1. A right shift is a DATE with CO2 • 2,3 Diphosphoglycerate DPG • Acidosis • Temperature • Exercise

O1. BATTED •Bathing •Ambulation •Toileting •Transfers •Eating •Dressing

P1. "CPR" • Compensatory Stage • Progressive Stage • Refractory Stage

Q1. CAMP • Condyloma lata • Acute Infection symptoms (fever, sore throat, malaise, weight loss) • Mucocutaneous lesion, mucous patches • Papules & Pustules

R1. CREAR: • Coronavirus • Rhinoviruses • Enterovirus •

___ 19. Walking Up and Down stairs with crutches

___ 20. Hisutism—The 5 Hs 5 Hs

___ 21. Hypoxia Symptoms: RAT BED

___ 22. Syphilis—Tertiary CLASS

___ 23. Liver Functions PUSH DoG

___ 24. White Blood Cells (In order of decreasing numbers.) "Nobody Likes My Educational Background" or "Never Let Monkeys Eat Bananas"

___ 25. heat vs cold first

___ 26. Nephritic Syndrome PHARAOH

___ 27. Teratogens TAP CAP

___ 28. Traction Care TRACTION

___ 29. Gestation—Bartholomew's Rule of Fours

___ 30. Cancer's Early Warning Signs CAUTION UP

___ 31. Prioritization The order in which we use the strategies in a priority question: PHAN

___ 32. Parkland Formula (Fluid Replacement) for Burns

___ 33. Esophageal Atresia and Tracheoesophageal Fistula 3 C's

___ 34. Sprains and Strains— Interventions RICE

___ 35. RUB MUB Compensation

___ 36. Triage color system Red, Yellow, Green, Black 32 can do

___ 37. Activities of Daily Living (ADL) BATTED

___ 38. Kidney Layers "Our Careers In Medicine"

___ 39. Intestinal Components Bowel Components (in order): Dow Jones Industrial Can't Choose Stocks

Adenovirus • Respiratory Syncytial Virus (RSV)

S1. A right shift is a DATE with CO2 •2,3 Diphosphoglycerate DPG •Acidosis •Temperature •Exercise

T1. RICE • Rest • Ice • Compression • Elevation

U1. "Rubber Ducky, I so Blue" • Rubella • Patent ductus arteriosus • Eyes • Blueberry muffin rash

V1. • 9% Head • 9% Chest • 9% Abdomen • 9% Upper back • 9% Lower back • 9% Anterior leg, each • 9% Posterior leg, each • 9% Entire arm, each • 1% Genitalia/perineum Rule of Palms: • 1% Palm of hand

W1. CN I: olfactory CN II: optic CN III: oculomotor CN IV: trochlear CN V: trigeminal CN VI: abducens CN VII: facial CN VIII: auditory or vestibulocochlear CN IX: glossopharyngeal CN X: vagus CN XI: spinal accessory CN XII: hypoglossal

X1. Red–Don't with within 15 mins they will die, ABC problem, above 30, no pulse, mentally confused Yellow–30 mins, not ABC but still wounded, above 30, pulse, mental status normal Green–emotional issues, walking wounded Black-dead, less 30 RR

Y1. P-S-E-U •Pneumonia •Sepsis •External otits media •UTI A-E-R-U-G-I-N-O-S-A •Aerobic •Exotoxin A •Rod •UTI, burns&infection •Green blue pigment •Iron containing lesions •Neg. gram,non lactose fermenting •Oxidase pos. •Sepsis •Adherence pili

Z1. S- I: olfactory S- II: optic M- III: oculomotor M- IV: trochlear B- V: trigeminal M- VI: abducens B- VII: facial S-VIII: auditory or vestibulocochlear B- IX: glossopharyngeal B- X: vagus M- XI: spinal accessory M- XII: hypoglossal

A2. PHARAOH • Proteinuria & Edema • Hematuria • Azotemia • RBC casts • Anti-strep titres (If post-strep) • Oliguria • Hypertension

B2. Sympathetic: fight or flight Parasympathetic: rest and digest

C2. •Change bowel/bladder •A lesion doesnt heal •Unusual bleeding/discharge •Thickening/lump breast/elsewhere •Indigestion/difficulty swallowing •Obvious change wart/mole •Nagging cough/persistent hoarseness •Unexplained weight loss •Pernicious Anemia

D2. E. coli causes DUNG • Diarrhea • UTI • Neonatal meningitis • Gram negative sepsis

E2. Gestation—Bartholomew's Rule of Fours • 12 Weeks: Symphisis pubis • 16 weeks: Midway between symphysis pubis and umbilicus • 20 weeks: Umbilicus • 36 weeks: Xiphoid process

F2. "HAVANA" • Hypovolemia • Adrenal Crisis • Vascular Stasis • Acute Respiratory Obstruction • Neurogenic • Anaphylaxis

G2. Hypothalamus wears TAN HATS • Thirst and water balance • Adenohypophysis • Neurohypophysis • Hunger and satiety

___ 40. Pseudomonas Aeruginosa
P-S-E-U & A-E-R-U-G-I-
N-O-S-A

___ 41. Syphilis—Secondary
CAMP

___ 42. The 5 A's of Alzheimers

___ 43. Acid-Base Balance ROME

___ 44. Hypothalamus Functions
Hypothalamus wears TAN
HATS

___ 45. Clubfoot—Deformities
InAdEquate

___ 46. Insulin Functions on Cells
INsulIN stimulates 2
things to go IN 2 cells:

___ 47. Scleroderma CREST
syndrome:

___ 48. Cranial nerves order "Oh,
oh, oh, to touch and feel a
girl's vagina. Such
heaven!"

___ 49. Dyspnea—Signs 6 Ps

___ 50. Common Cold—Causes
CREAR:

___ 51. Shock—Causes
"HAVANA"

___ 52. Oxygen Dissociation—
Right Shift A right shift is
a DATE with CO2

___ 53. Canes and Walkers COAL
and WWAL

___ 54. Cranial nerves : S: sensory;
m: motor; b: both "Some
say marry money but my
brother says big brains
matter more"

___ 55. Melanoma Characteristics
ABCDE

___ 56. PROM vs. PPROM

___ 57. Nursing Process How to
find the correct answer by
using the nursing process.
Assess before you
implement! ADPIE:

___ 58. Decels and Accels (FHR)
Change> Cause> What to
do VEAL >CHOP> MINE

___ 59. Streptococcus pyogenes—

• Autonomic regulation • Temperature regulation • Sexual
urges and emotions

H2. GET NIPPLES • Glomerulonephritis • Endocarditis (Heart
Valves) • Toxic shock syndrome • Necrotizing fasciitis and
myositis • Impetigo • Pharyngitis • Pneumonia •
Lymphangitis • Erysipelas and cellulitis • Scarlet
fever/Rheumatic Fever

I2. 5 Hs • Hirsutism • Hyperplasia of gums • Harm to kidneys •
Hypertension • Hyperglycemia

J2. I-SBAR: •Identify •Situation •Background •Assessment
•Recommendation

K2. Variable Dec>Cord
compression>Move(Trendelenburg>Csection) Early
Dec>Head Compression>Identify Labor(active good, no
progression bad) Accel>OK>Nothing Late Dec>Placenta
Insufficiency>Execute actions NOW (move, turn off Pitocin,
^fluids, O2, Csection)

L2. ABCDE • Asymmetrical • Borders irregular • Color dark and
variation • Diameter is large (> 6MM) • Evolving

M2. FROM JANE • Fever • Roth's spots • Osler's nodes •
Murmur • Janeway lesions • Anemia • Nail hemorrhage
(splinter hemorrhages) • Emboli

N2. COAL • Cane • Opposite • Affected • Leg WWAL • Walker •
With • Affected • Leg

O2. Use heat first for muscles Use cold first for nerves

P2. Kidney layers "Our Careers In Medicine" • Outer cortex •
Inner medulla

Q2. [4 x wgt (kg) x TBSA %] / 2 = ANSWER ANSWER – give
in first 8 hours ANSWER – give in next 16 hours

R2. ABCDE secondary causes • Aldosterone/Apnea • Bad
kidney/Bruits • Catecholamines/Cushings syndrome •
Drugs/Diet • Endocrine

S2. AIDS—The Cells Attacked AIDS is 4 letters long. AIDS
attacks CD4 T cells.

T2. CLASS • Cardiovascular disorder • Late benign syphilis
(gumma) • Asymptomatic Neurosyphilis • Symptomatic
Neurosyphilis • Seizures and apathy (signs of meningeal
involvement)

U2. CREST syndrome: • Calcinosis • Raynaud's Syndrome •
Esophageal Motility Disorder • Sclerodactyly •
Telangiectasia

V2. SCUM •Shopping •Cooking and Cleaning •Using telephone
or transportation •Managing money and medications

W2. Good people go to heaven (good leg up) Bad people go to
hell (bad leg down)

X2. RAT BED • Early Hypoxia: Restlessness Anxiety
Tachycardia/ Tachypnea • Late Hypoxia: Bradycardia
Extreme Restlessness Dyspnea

Diseases GET NIPPLES

___ 60. Shock—Stages "CPR"

___ 61. Hypertension—Causes
Use the ABCDE method to
identify secondary causes.

___ 62. Risk factors for primary
hypertension: SOSAD IC

___ 63. Instrumental Activities of
Daily Living (IADL)
SCUM

___ 64. Naegele's rule

___ 65. Oxygen Dissociation—
Right Shift A right shift is
a DATE with CO2

___ 66. Hypoglycemia TIRED

___ 67. AIDS—The Cells
Attacked

___ 68. Burns—Rule of Nines and
Rule of Palms Total body
surface area (TBSA): Rule
of Nines:

Y2. ROME Respiratory Opposite • pH up PCO2 down =
Alkalosis • pH down PCO2 up = Acidosis Metabolic Equal •
pH up HCO3 up = Alkalosis • pH down HCO3 down =
Acidosis

Z2. •Neutrophils •Lymphocytes •Monocytes •Eosinophils ·
•Basophils

A3. Staph aureus caused by SOFT PAINS • Skin infections •
Osteomyelitis • Food poisoning • Toxic shock syndrome •
Pneumonia • Acute endocarditis • Infective arthritis •
Necrotizing fasciitis • Sepsis

B3. 1. Amnesia (memory loss) 2. Anomia (unable to recall
names of objects) 3. Apraxia (inability to perform particular
purposive actions) 4. Agonsia (inability to interpret
sensations & recognize things) 5. Aphasia (inability to
understand/express speech)

C3. Assess before you implement! ADPIE: •Assessment
•Diagnosis •Planning •Implementation •Evaluation

D3. Flow of fluid "Be Prepared To Look Happy During
Computer-based Testing" •Bowmans capsule •Proximal
Tubules •Loop Henle •Distal and Convoluted Tubules

E3. PUSH DoG • Protein synthesis • Ureas synthesis • Storage •
Hormone synthesis • Detoxification • Glucose and fat
metabolism

F3. D.I.G. F.A.S.T. Distractibility Indiscretion Grandiosity Flight
of Ideas Activity Increase Sleep Deficit Talkative

G3. CRAB: • Calcium level elevated • Renal failure • Anemia •
Bone breakdown and resorption

H3. InAdEquate • Inversion • Adduction • Equinus

I3. 6 Ps •Pneumonia •Pulmonary Bronchial Constriction
•Possible Foreign Body •Pulmonary Embolus •Pneumothorax
•Pump Failure

J3. Hormones that Increase Blood Glucose "STENGG" •
Somatotropin (growth hormone) • Thyroid hormones
(thyroxine and triiodothyronine) • Epinephrine •
Norepinephrine • Glucagon • Glucocorticosteroids

K3. Respiratory Uses Bicarb, Metabolic Uses Breathing •
Respiratory Acidosis, Retain Bicarb • Respiratory Alkalosis,
Excrete Bicarb • Metabolic Acidosis, Increase Breathing •
Metabolic Alkalosis, Decrease Breathing

L3. PRISH • Pain • Redness • Immobility (loss of function) •
Swelling • Heat

M3. SOSAD IC •Sodium and fat intake •Obesity •Stress
•Alcohol •D vitamin deficiency •Inactivity •Caffeine

N3. People Have Endless Appetites • Proteinuria •
Hyperlipidemia • Edema • Albuminuria & hypoalbuminemia

O3. INsulIN stimulates 2 things to go IN 2 cells: Potassium and
Glucose.

P3. 1. Getting ready to Push a. Latent – 0-3, little to no pain b.

Active – 3-7, c. Transition – 7-10, effacement 100% 2. Pushing = Baby 3. Placenta 4. Bonding

Mnemonics
Quiz and Test

Nursing Mnemonics Quiz

Circle the letter of the Answer that corresponds to the displayed Question.

1. Severe Pre-Eclampsia (HELLP)

    A. H- emolysis E- levated L- iver function tests L- ow P- latelet count

    B. D-elirium I-nfection A-trophic Urethra P-harmaceuticals P-sychologic E-xcess Urine Output R-estricted Mobility S-tool Impaction

    C. W- Walker W- With A- Affected L - Leg

    D. C- Choking C- Coughing C - Cyanosis

2. CANCER'S Early Warning Signs CAUTION UP

    A. S-lurred Speech A-ltered Central Nervous System M-uscle Twitching S-eizures

    B. Change in bowel/bladder A lesion doesn't heal Unusual bleeding/discharge Thickening lump in breast/elsewhere Indigestion/difficulty swallowing Obvious changes wart/mole Nagging cough/persistent hoarseness Unexplained weight loss Pernicious Anemia

    C. M - Muscle weakness U - Urine, oliguria, anuria R- Respiratory distress D - Decreased cardiac contractility E - ECG changes R - Reflexes, hyperreflexia, or areflexia (flaccid)

    D. Amenorrhea delayed No organic factors accounts for weight loss Obviously thin but feels FAT Refusal to maintain normal body weight Epigastric discomfort is common Xsymptoms (peculiar symptoms) Intense fears of gaining weight Always thinking of foods

3. Immediate Treatment of a Myocardial Infarction Client (MONA)

    A. M- Morphine O- Oxygen N- Nitroglycerine A- ASA

    B. D- Denial D- Dependency D- Demanding D- Destructive D- Domineering

    C. D- Distractibility I - Indiscretion G - Grandiosity F- Flight of Ideas A- Activity Increase S- Sleep Deficit T - Talkative

    D. F- Frequency U- Urgency N- Nocturia

4. Nursing Care for Sprains and Strains (RICE)

    A. A-drenergics (Albuterol) S-teroids T-heophylline H-ydration (IV) M-ask (Oxygen) A-ntibiotics

    B. F - Frequency (3x per week) I - Intensity (60-80% of Maximal Heart Rate) T- Time (Aerobic Activity)

    C. R- Rest I - Ice C - Compression E- Elevation

    D. P- Polyuria (excessive urination) P- Polydypsia (excessive thirst) P- Polyphagia (excessive hunger)

5. Cranial Nerve Mnemonic 02

    A. A-irway B-reathing C-irculation D-isability E-xamine F-ahrenheit G-et Vitals H-ead to Toe Assessment I-ntervention

    B. O- Oh O- Oh O- Oh T- To T- Touch A- And F - Feel A G - irl's V - agina S - So H- Heavenly

    C. C-oncentration decreased A-ppetite P-sychomotor function decreased S-uicidal Ideations

    D. S-lurred Speech A-ltered Central Nervous System M-uscle Twitching S-eizures

6. Emergency Drugs to LEAN on

    A. L- Lidocaine E - Epinephrine A- Atropine Sulfate N - Narcan

    B. C-omfort A-ltered Body Image N-utrition C-hemotherapy E-valuate response to meds R-espite for caretakers

C. F-eeding difficulty I-nspiratory Stridor N-ares Flares E-xpiratory Grunting S-ternal Retractions

D. S-lurred Speech A-ltered Central Nervous System M-uscle Twitching S-eizures

7. Trauma Surgery (AMPLE) after initial assessment

A. A-llergies M-edications P-ast Medical History L-ast Meal E-vents Surrounding Injury

B. Early Hypoxia: R-estlessness A-nxiety T-achycardia/ Tachypnea Late Hypoxia: B-radycardia E-xtreme Restlessness D-yspnea

C. N - Non-reactive N - Non- Stress is N - Not good

D. Make sure they don't have problems with: D-rug and alcohol E-yes and ears M-etabolic and endocrine disorders E-motional disorders N-eurologic disorders T-umors and trauma I-nfection A-rteriovascular disease

8. Treating CHF (UNLOAD FAST)

A. A-ssessment A-nanlysis P-lanning I-mplementation E-valuation

B. U-pright Position N-itrates (in low dose) L-asix O-xygen A-minophylline D-igoxin F-luids (decrease) A-fterload (decrease) S-odium restriction T-est (Dig level, ABGs, K level)

C. Child's excessive knowledge on sex & abusive words Hair growth in various lengths Inconsistent stories from the child & parent/s Low self-esteem Depression Apathy, no emotion Bruised Unusual injuries Serious injuries Evidence of old injuries not reported

D. D-elirium I-nfection A-trophic Urethra P-harmaceuticals P-sychologic E-xcess Urine Output R-estricted Mobility S-tool Impaction

9. To apply a telemetry monitor:

A. White over right (top right shoulder) Black beside the white (Over lt shoulder) Checkers (red below the black) Christmas (Green beside the red) Then ofcourse, the brown will be in the middle!

B. B-reasts U-terus B-owels B-ladder L-ochia E-pisiotomy/lateration/C-section incision

C. T-ricuspid P-ulmonic M-itrial A-ortic

D. W- Walker W- With A- Affected L - Leg

10. Evalution of Episiotomy Healing (REEDA)

A. N - Non-reactive N - Non- Stress is N - Not good

B. T-achycardia I-rritability R-estless E-xcessive Hunger D-iaphoresis/ Depression

C. A-mnesia A-nomia A-praxia A-gnosia A-phasia

D. R- Redness E- Edema E - Ecchymosis D - Discharge, Drainage A - Approximation

Circle the letter of the Question that corresponds to the displayed Answer.

11. F - Frequency (3x per week) I - Intensity (60-80% of Maximal Heart Rate) T- Time (Aerobic Activity)

A. Evalution of Episiotomy Healing (REEDA)

B. Steps in the Nursing Process ADPIE (A Delicious PIE)

C. Lidocaine Toxicity (SAMS)

D. Exercise Guide for Diabetic Fitness (FIT)

12. C- Coronary Artery Disease C- Coronary Rheumatic Fever C- Congestive Heart Failure C- Cardio Vascular Accident

A. Osteoporosis Risk Factors (ACCESS)

B. Acid-Base (ROME)

C. Symptoms of Hypoxia (RAT BED)

D. 4 C's of Hypertension (Complications)

13. F - Fever (low grade), flushed skin R - Restless (irritable) I - Increased fluid retention and increased BP E - Edema (peripheral and pitting) D - Decreased urinary output, dry mouth

    A. Inflammation (HIPER)

    B. Nursing Care for Sprains and Strains (RICE)

    C. Drugs for Bradycardia & low BP (IDEA)

    D. HYPERNATREMIA "You Are Fried"

14. OLympic (Olfactory) OPium (Optic) OCcupies (Oculomotor) TROubled (Trochlear) TRIathletes (Trigeminal) After (Abducens) Finishing (Facial) VEgas (Vestibulocochlear) Gambling (Glossopharyngeal) VAcations (Vagus) Still (Spinal Accessory) High (Hypoglossal)

    A. Prostate Problems are no... FUN

    B. Cranial Nerve Mnemonic 01

    C. Anticholingergics Side Effects: 4-CAN'Ts

    D. Energy Decreased (CAPS)

15. P- Preventable P- Painless P- Permanent

    A. Evalution of Episiotomy Healing (REEDA)

    B. Depression Assessment (SIG)

    C. 3 P's of Blindness

    D. Steps in the Nursing Process AAPIE (An Apple Pie)

16. C - Convulsions A- Arrhythmias T - Tetany S - Spasms and stridor

    A. "CATS" of "HYPOCALCEMIA"

    B. To apply a telemetry monitor:

    C. MI management: MONA

    D. Prostate Problems are no... FUN

17. R-espiratory O-pposite M-etabolic E-qual

    A. ADLs (Activity of Daily Living) BATTED

    B. Acid-Base (ROME)

    C. Lidocaine Toxicity (SAMS)

    D. TDCI (These Drugs Can Interact)

18. W- Walker W- With A- Affected L - Leg

    A. Canes and Walkers (WWAL) Wandering Wilma's Always Late

    B. Major Symptoms of a Manic Attack (DIG FAST)

    C. Trauma Surgery (AMPLE) after initial assessment

    D. TDCI (These Drugs Can Interact)

19. P- Pulmonary Bronchial Constriction P- Possible Foreign Body P- Pulmonary Embolus P- Pneumothorax P- Pump Failure P- Pneumonia

A. 6 P's of Dyspnea

B. Treating CHF (UNLOAD FAST)

C. CANCER'S Early Warning Signs CAUTION UP

D. Common Causes of Transient Incontinence (DIAPPERS)

20. A-llergies M-edications P-ast Medical History L-ast Meal E-vents Surrounding Injury

A. Hyperkalemia Management (KIND)

B. Promotion of Normal Elimination (POOPER SCOOP)

C. Trauma Surgery (AMPLE) after initial assessment

D. Energy Decreased (CAPS)

EXTRA CREDIT: Give the Question that corresponds to the displayed Answer.

21. Make sure they don't have problems with: D-rug and alcohol E-yes and ears M-etabolic and endocrine disorders E-motional disorders N-eurologic disorders T-umors and trauma I-nfection A-rteriovascular disease

Mnemonics for NCLEX Quiz

Circle the letter of the Answer that corresponds to the displayed Question.

1. Autonomic Nervous System Functions Rhyme

    A. Sympathetic: fight or flight Parasympathetic: rest and digest

    B. Kidney layers "Our Careers In Medicine" • Outer cortex • Inner medulla

    C. SCUM •Shopping •Cooking and Cleaning •Using telephone or transportation •Managing money and medications

    D. I-SBAR: •Identify •Situation •Background •Assessment •Recommendation

2. Instrumental Activities of Daily Living (IADL) SCUM

    A. [4 x wgt (kg) x TBSA %] / 2 = ANSWER ANSWER – give in first 8 hours ANSWER – give in next 16 hours

    B. BATTED •Bathing •Ambulation •Toileting •Transfers •Eating •Dressing

    C. SCUM •Shopping •Cooking and Cleaning •Using telephone or transportation •Managing money and medications

    D. People Have Endless Appetites • Proteinuria • Hyperlipidemia • Edema • Albuminuria & hypoalbuminemia

3. Nephritic Syndrome PHARAOH

    A. PHARAOH • Proteinuria & Edema • Hematuria • Azotemia • RBC casts • Anti-strep titres (If post-strep) • Oliguria • Hypertension

    B. ABCDE • Asymmetrical • Borders irregular • Color dark and variation • Diameter is large (> 6MM) • Evolving

    C. I-SBAR: •Identify •Situation •Background •Assessment •Recommendation

    D. CN I: olfactory CN II: optic CN III: oculomotor CN IV: trochlear CN V: trigeminal CN VI: abducens CN VII: facial CN VIII: auditory or vestibulocochlear CN IX: glossopharyngeal CN X: vagus CN XI: spinal accessory CN XII: hypoglossal

4. Cancer's Early Warning Signs CAUTION UP

    A. TAP CAP • Thalidomide • Alcohol • Progestins • Corticosteroids • Aspirin • Phenytoin

    B. "HAVANA" • Hypovolemia • Adrenal Crisis • Vascular Stasis • Acute Respiratory Obstruction • Neurogenic • Anaphylaxis

    C. •Change bowel/bladder •A lesion doesnt heal •Unusual bleeding/discharge •Thickening/lump breast/elsewhere •Indigestion/difficulty swallowing •Obvious change wart/mole •Nagging cough/persistent hoarseness •Unexplained weight loss •Pernicious Anemia

    D. TIRED • Tachycardia • Irritability • Restlessness • Excessive Hunger • Diaphoresis Rhyme Cold and clammy, need some candy

5. Prioritization The order in which we use the strategies in a priority question: PHAN

    A. Gestation—Bartholomew's Rule of Fours • 12 Weeks: Symphisis pubis • 16 weeks: Midway between symphysis pubis and umbilicus • 20 weeks: Umbilicus • 36 weeks: Xiphoid process

    B. CREAR: • Coronavirus • Rhinoviruses • Enterovirus • Adenovirus • Respiratory Syncytial Virus (RSV)

    C. SCUM •Shopping •Cooking and Cleaning •Using telephone or transportation •Managing money and medications

    D. PHAN •Priority •Hierarchy •ABCs •Nursing Process

6. Dyspnea—Signs 6 Ps

A. Use heat first for muscles Use cold first for nerves

B. RAT BED • Early Hypoxia: Restlessness Anxiety Tachycardia/ Tachypnea • Late Hypoxia: Bradycardia Extreme Restlessness Dyspnea

C. Gestation—Bartholomew's Rule of Fours • 12 Weeks: Symphisis pubis • 16 weeks: Midway between symphysis pubis and umbilicus • 20 weeks: Umbilicus • 36 weeks: Xiphoid process

D. 6 Ps •Pneumonia •Pulmonary Bronchial Constriction •Possible Foreign Body •Pulmonary Embolus •Pneumothorax •Pump Failure

7. Walking Up and Down stairs with crutches

A. AIDS—The Cells Attacked AIDS is 4 letters long. AIDS attacks CD4 T cells.

B. SOSAD IC •Sodium and fat intake •Obesity •Stress •Alcohol •D vitamin deficiency •Inactivity •Caffeine

C. Good people go to heaven (good leg up) Bad people go to hell (bad leg down)

D. "HAVANA" • Hypovolemia • Adrenal Crisis • Vascular Stasis • Acute Respiratory Obstruction • Neurogenic • Anaphylaxis

8. Hyperglycemia 3 P's

A. Flow of fluid "Be Prepared To Look Happy During Computer-based Testing" •Bowmans capsule •Proximal Tubules •Loop Henle •Distal and Convoluted Tubules

B. 3 P's • Polyphagia • Polydipsia • Polyuria Rhyme Hot and dry, sugar high

C. People Have Endless Appetites • Proteinuria • Hyperlipidemia • Edema • Albuminuria & hypoalbuminemia

D. "HAVANA" • Hypovolemia • Adrenal Crisis • Vascular Stasis • Acute Respiratory Obstruction • Neurogenic • Anaphylaxis

9. Oxygen Dissociation—Right Shift A right shift is a DATE with CO2

A. A right shift is a DATE with CO2 •2,3 Diphosphoglycerate DPG •Acidosis •Temperature •Exercise

B. Rubra (3-5 days, blood & clots) Serosa (10 days, pink) Alba (up to 2-5 weeks, Should not be longer than 6 weeks, white/creamy)

C. AIDS—The Cells Attacked AIDS is 4 letters long. AIDS attacks CD4 T cells.

D. TRACTION • Temperature (Extremity, Infection) • hang freely • Alignment • Circulation Check (5 P's) • Type & Location of fracture • Increase fluide intake • Overhead trapeze • No weights on bed or floor

10. Nursing Process How to find the correct answer by using the nursing process. Assess before you implement! ADPIE:

A. Assess before you implement! ADPIE: •Assessment •Diagnosis •Planning •Implementation •Evaluation

B. Use heat first for muscles Use cold first for nerves

C. Sympathetic: fight or flight Parasympathetic: rest and digest

D. Staph aureus caused by SOFT PAINS • Skin infections • Osteomyelitis • Food poisoning • Toxic shock syndrome • Pneumonia • Acute endocarditis • Infective arthritis • Necrotizing fasciitis • Sepsis

Circle the letter of the Question that corresponds to the displayed Answer.

11. TAP CAP • Thalidomide • Alcohol • Progestins • Corticosteroids • Aspirin • Phenytoin

A. Nephrotic Syndrome People Have Endless Appetites

B. Teratogens TAP CAP

C. PROM vs. PPROM

D. Risk factors for primary hypertension: SOSAD IC

12. Kidney layers "Our Careers In Medicine" • Outer cortex • Inner medulla

    A. Dyspnea—Signs 6 Ps

    B. Kidney Layers "Our Careers In Medicine"

    C. Syphilis—Secondary CAMP

    D. Hyperglycemia 3 P's

13. TIRED • Tachycardia • Irritability • Restlessness • Excessive Hunger • Diaphoresis Rhyme Cold and clammy, need some candy

    A. Nursing Process How to find the correct answer by using the nursing process. Assess before you implement! ADPIE:

    B. Parkland Formula (Fluid Replacement) for Burns

    C. Hypoglycemia TIRED

    D. AIDS—The Cells Attacked

14. PRISH • Pain • Redness • Immobility (loss of function) • Swelling • Heat

    A. Hyperglycemia 3 P's

    B. Insulin Functions on Cells INsulIN stimulates 2 things to go IN 2 cells:

    C. Inflammation—Signs PRISH

    D. RUB MUB Compensation

15. 1. Amnesia (memory loss) 2. Anomia (unable to recall names of objects) 3. Apraxia (inability to perform particular purposive actions) 4. Agonsia (inability to interpret sensations & recognize things) 5. Aphasia (inability to understand/express speech)

    A. The 5 A's of Alzheimers

    B. Dyspnea—Signs 6 Ps

    C. Risk factors for primary hypertension: SOSAD IC

    D. Common Cold—Causes CREAR:

16. Dow Jones Industrial Can't Choose Stocks • Duodenum • Jejunum • Ileum • Cecum • Colon • Sigmoid

    A. Patient Handoff Report I-SBAR patient handoff reporting supports the National Patient Safety Goal #2, "to improve effectiveness of communication among caregivers."

    B. Activities of Daily Living (ADL) BATTED

    C. Intestinal Components Bowel Components (in order): Dow Jones Industrial Can't Choose Stocks

    D. Sprains and Strains—Interventions RICE

17. [4 x wgt (kg) x TBSA %] / 2 = ANSWER ANSWER – give in first 8 hours ANSWER – give in next 16 hours

    A. Flow of fluid through the Kidney "Be Prepared To Look Happy During Computer-based Testing"

    B. Pseudomonas Aeruginosa P-S-E-U & A-E-R-U-G-I-N-O-S-A

    C. Liver Functions PUSH DoG

    D. Parkland Formula (Fluid Replacement) for Burns

18. Hormones that Increase Blood Glucose "STENGG" • Somatotropin (growth hormone) • Thyroid hormones (thyroxine and triiodothyronine) • Epinephrine • Norepinephrine • Glucagon •

Glucocorticosteroids

    A. Shock—Causes "HAVANA"

    B. Postpartum Lochia changes

    C. Cancer's Early Warning Signs CAUTION UP

    D. Blood Glucose—Hormonal Influence Hormones that Increase Blood Glucose "STENGG"

19. People Have Endless Appetites • Proteinuria • Hyperlipidemia • Edema • Albuminuria & hypoalbuminemia

    A. Walking Up and Down stairs with crutches

    B. Instrumental Activities of Daily Living (IADL) SCUM

    C. Nephrotic Syndrome People Have Endless Appetites

    D. heat vs cold first

20. Rubra (3-5 days, blood & clots) Serosa (10 days, pink) Alba (up to 2-5 weeks, Should not be longer than 6 weeks, white/creamy)

    A. Nephritic Syndrome PHARAOH

    B. White Blood Cells (In order of decreasing numbers.) "Nobody Likes My Educational Background" or "Never Let Monkeys Eat Bananas"

    C. Postpartum Lochia changes

    D. Rubella, Congenital—Signs "Rubber Ducky, I so Blue"

Nursing Mnemonics Test

Enter the letter for the matching Answer

1. ☐ Cholinergic Crisis (SLUD)
2. ☐ 3 P's of Diabetes Mellitus - Type 1 Signs & Symptoms
3. ☐ Eating Disorder: BULIMIA
4. ☐ CANCER'S Early Warning Signs CAUTION UP
5. ☐ DEMENTIA
6. ☐ Acid-Base (ROME)
7. ☐ Serious Complications of Oral Birth Control Pills (ACHES)
8. ☐ Situations requiring Crisis Situation: RAPE
9. ☐ 5 A's to Alzheimer Diagnosis
10. ☐ Gluten Free Diet (ROW)
11. ☐ Right-Sided Heart Failure (HEAD)
12. ☐ MI management: MONA
13. ☐ Anticholingergics Side Effects: 4-CAN'Ts
14. ☐ HYPOGLYCEMIA: TIRED
15. ☐ Lidocaine Toxicity (SAMS)
16. ☐ Pulmonary Edema (MAD DOG)
17. ☐ ADLs (Activity of Daily Living) BATTED
18. ☐ Steps in the Nursing Process ADPIE (A Delicious PIE)

A. A- Abdominal Pain C - Chest Pain H - Headache E - Eye Problems S - Severe Leg Pain

B. S-lurred Speech A-ltered Central Nervous System M-uscle Twitching S-eizures

C. H- Hepatomegaly E- Edema (Bipedal) A- Ascites D- Distended Neck Vein

D. P- Polyuria (excessive urination) P- Polydypsia (excessive thirst) P- Polyphagia (excessive hunger)

E. A-ssessment D- iagnosis P-lanning I-mplementation E-valuaton

F. R-espiratory O-pposite M-etabolic E-qual

G. Make sure they don't have problems with: D-rug and alcohol E-yes and ears M-etabolic and endocrine disorders E-motional disorders N-eurologic disorders T-umors and trauma I-nfection A-rteriovascular disease

H. Can't see Can't pee Can't spit Can't sh*t

I. R- Rye O- Oats W- Wheat

J. T Tired I Irritability R Restless E Excessive hunger D Diaphoresis-Depression

K. S-alivation L-acrimation U-rination D-efecation

L. M-Morphine A-Aminophylline D- Digitalis D-Diuretics (Lasix) O- Oxygen G- ases (Blood Gases ABG's)

M. B- Banana R- Rice A- Apple T- Toasted Bread

N. Change in bowel/bladder A lesion doesn't heal Unusual bleeding/discharge Thickening lump in breast/elsewhere Indigestion/difficulty swallowing Obvious changes wart/mole Nagging cough/persistent hoarseness Unexplained weight loss Pernicious Anemia

O. Morphine O2 Nitroglycerine Aspirin

P. R- Ruthless A- Abusive P- Personal E- Experience

Q. A-mnesia A-nomia A-praxia A-gnosia A-phasia

R. S-hopping C-ooking and Cleaning U-sing telephone or transportaiton M-anaging money and medications

S. B-inge eating U-nder strict dieting L-acks control over-eating I-nduced vomiting M-inimum of to binge eating episodes I-ncrease/Persistent concern of body size/shape A-buse of diuretics & laxatives

T. B-athing A-mbulation T-oileting T-ransfers E-ating D-ressing

19. ☐ IADLS
    (Instrumental
    Activities of Daily
    Living) SCUM

20. ☐ BRAT Diet (for
    severe
    dehydration)

Give the Question that corresponds to the displayed Answer.

21. P- Potassium I- Inside S- Sodium O- Outside

22. C - Convulsions A- Arrhythmias T - Tetany S - Spasms and stridor

23. C-oncentration decreased A-ppetite P-sychomotor function decreased S-uicidal Ideations

24. Amenorrhea delayed No organic factors accounts for weight loss Obviously thin but feels FAT Refusal to maintain normal body weight Epigastric discomfort is common Xsymptoms (peculiar symptoms) Intense fears of gaining weight Always thinking of foods

25. H-eat I-nduration P-ain E-dema R-edness

26. S Stenosis P Partial obstruction A Aneurysms S Septal defect M Mitral regurgitation

27. A-irway Closed I-ncreased Pulse R-estlessness R-etractions A-nxiety Increased I-nspiratory Stridor D-rooling

28. C-omfort A-ltered Body Image N-utrition C-hemotherapy E-valuate response to meds R-espite for caretakers

29. S-lurred Speech A-ltered Central Nervous System M-uscle Twitching S-eizures

30. A-drenergics (Albuterol) S-teroids T-heophylline H-ydration (IV) M-ask (Oxygen) A-ntibiotics

Mnemonics for NCLEX Test

Enter the letter for the matching Answer

1. ☐ PROM vs. PPROM

2. ☐ Liver Functions PUSH DoG

3. ☐ Melanoma Characteristics ABCDE

4. ☐ Decels and Accels (FHR) Change> Cause> What to do VEAL >CHOP> MINE

5. ☐ Prioritization The order in which we use the strategies in a priority question: PHAN

6. ☐ Kidney Layers "Our Careers In Medicine"

7. ☐ Asthma Management ASTHMA:

8. ☐ RUB MUB Compensation

9. ☐ Cancer's Early Warning Signs CAUTION UP

10. ☐ Streptococcus pyogenes— Diseases GET NIPPLES

11. ☐ Triage color system Red, Yellow, Green, Black 32 can do

12. ☐ Blood Glucose —Hormonal Influence Hormones that Increase Blood Glucose "STENGG"

A. PHAN •Priority •Hierarchy •ABCs •Nursing Process

B. PHARAOH • Proteinuria & Edema • Hematuria • Azotemia • RBC casts • Anti-strep titres (If post-strep) • Oliguria • Hypertension

C. Staph aureus caused by SOFT PAINS • Skin infections • Osteomyelitis • Food poisoning • Toxic shock syndrome • Pneumonia • Acute endocarditis • Infective arthritis • Necrotizing fasciitis • Sepsis

D. Variable Dec>Cord compression>Move(Trendelenburg>Csection) Early Dec>Head Compression>Identify Labor(active good, no progression bad) Accel>OK>Nothing Late Dec>Placenta Insufficiency>Execute actions NOW (move, turn off Pitocin, ^fluids, O2, Csection)

E. 1. Getting ready to Push a. Latent – 0-3, little to no pain b. Active – 3-7, c. Transition – 7-10, effacement 100% 2. Pushing = Baby 3. Placenta 4. Bonding

F. GET NIPPLES • Glomerulonephritis • Endocarditis (Heart Valves) • Toxic shock syndrome • Necrotizing fasciitis and myositis • Impetigo • Pharyngitis • Pneumonia • Lymphangitis • Erysipelas and cellulitis • Scarlet fever/Rheumatic Fever

G. ABCDE • Asymmetrical • Borders irregular • Color dark and variation • Diameter is large (> 6MM) • Evolving

H. *PROM(Premature Rupture of Membrane) = More than 1 hour before onset of labor, Use Pitocin to get things moving *PPROM (Preterm)= 37 weeks and More than 1 hour before onset of labor, Risk for infection (prophylactic ATB), Bed Rest, Steroids (if needed)

I. D.I.G. F.A.S.T. Distractibility Indiscretion Grandiosity Flight of Ideas Activity Increase Sleep Deficit Talkative

J. Hormones that Increase Blood Glucose "STENGG" • Somatotropin (growth hormone) • Thyroid hormones (thyroxine and triiodothyronine) • Epinephrine • Norepinephrine • Glucagon • Glucocorticosteroids

K. Red–Don't with within 15 mins they will die, ABC problem, above 30, no pulse, mentally confused Yellow–30 mins, not ABC but still wounded, above 30, pulse, mental status normal Green–emotional issues, walking wounded Black-dead, less 30 RR

L. FROM JANE • Fever • Roth's spots • Osler's nodes • Murmur • Janeway lesions • Anemia • Nail hemorrhage (splinter hemorrhages) • Emboli

M. Good people go to heaven (good leg up) Bad people go to hell (bad leg down)

N. CN I: olfactory CN II: optic CN III: oculomotor CN IV: trochlear CN V: trigeminal CN VI: abducens CN VII: facial CN VIII: auditory or

13. ☐ Staph aureus caused by SOFT PAINS

14. ☐ Cranial nerves order "Oh, oh, oh, to touch and feel a girl's vagina. Such heaven!"

15. ☐ Stages of Labor

16. ☐ Patient Handoff Report I-SBAR patient handoff reporting supports the National Patient Safety Goal #2, "to improve effectiveness of communication among caregivers."

17. ☐ Nephritic Syndrome PHARAOH

18. ☐ Endocarditis signs FROM JANE

19. ☐ Bipolar Mania Symptoms

20. ☐ Walking Up and Down stairs with crutches

vestibulocochlear CN IX: glossopharyngeal CN X: vagus CN XI: spinal accessory CN XII: hypoglossal

O. Kidney layers "Our Careers In Medicine" • Outer cortex • Inner medulla

P. I-SBAR: •Identify •Situation •Background •Assessment •Recommendation

Q. ASTHMA: •Adrenergics (Albuterol) •Steroids •Theophylline •Hydration (IV) •Mask (Oxygen) •Antibiotics (Infection)

R. Respiratory Uses Bicarb, Metabolic Uses Breathing • Respiratory Acidosis, Retain Bicarb • Respiratory Alkalosis, Excrete Bicarb • Metabolic Acidosis, Increase Breathing • Metabolic Alkalosis, Decrease Breathing

S. •Change bowel/bladder •A lesion doesnt heal •Unusual bleeding/discharge •Thickening/lump breast/elsewhere •Indigestion/difficulty swallowing •Obvious change wart/mole •Nagging cough/persistent hoarseness •Unexplained weight loss •Pernicious Anemia

T. PUSH DoG • Protein synthesis • Ureas synthesis • Storage • Hormone synthesis • Detoxification • Glucose and fat metabolism

Give the Question that corresponds to the displayed Answer.

21. TAP CAP • Thalidomide • Alcohol • Progestins • Corticosteroids • Aspirin • Phenytoin

22. Rubra (3-5 days, blood & clots) Serosa (10 days, pink) Alba (up to 2-5 weeks, Should not be longer than 6 weeks, white/creamy)

23. 6 Ps •Pneumonia •Pulmonary Bronchial Constriction •Possible Foreign Body •Pulmonary Embolus •Pneumothorax •Pump Failure

24. "HAVANA" • Hypovolemia • Adrenal Crisis • Vascular Stasis • Acute Respiratory Obstruction • Neurogenic • Anaphylaxis

25. "CPR" • Compensatory Stage • Progressive Stage • Refractory Stage

26. CLASS • Cardiovascular disorder • Late benign syphilis (gumma) • Asymptomatic Neurosyphilis • Symptomatic Neurosyphilis • Seizures and apathy (signs of meningeal involvement)

27. PRESS • Painless lesion • Regional lymphadenopathy • Exudate • Single lesion • Sexual contact can cause

28. CAMP • Condyloma lata • Acute Infection symptoms (fever, sore throat, malaise, weight loss) • Mucocutaneous lesion, mucous patches • Papules & Pustules

29. TRACTION • Temperature (Extremity, Infection) • hang freely • Alignment • Circulation Check (5 P's) • Type & Location of fracture • Increase fluide intake • Overhead trapeze • No weights on bed or floor

30. 1st day of LMP - 3 months (don't forget to adjust year if needed) + 7 days (don't forget to adjust the month if needed)